INJURY REHAB

with

RESISTANCE BANDS

COMPLETE ANATOMICAL
INFORMATION AND REHABILITATION
ROUTINES FOR BACK, NECK,
SHOULDERS, ELBOWS, HIPS, KNEES,
ANKLES AND MORE

DR. KARL KNOPF

CHRIS KNOPF, ADVISOR

 ULYSSES PRESS

Published in the United States by
Ulysses Press
PO Box 3440
Berkeley, CA 94703
www.ulyssespress.com

ISBN: 978-1-61243-449-0
Library of Congress Control Number: 2014952007

Printed in the United States
10 9 8 7 6 5 4 3

Acquisitions: Kelly Reed
Managing editor: Claire Chun
Project editor: Lindsay Tamura
Editor: Lily Chou
Proofreader: Renee Rutledge
Indexer: Sayre Van Young
Front cover/interior design: what!design @ whatweb.com
Front cover photographs: woman © Doruk Sikman/shutterstock.com; starburst © FMStox/shutterstock.com
Back cover photographs: © Rapt Productions
Models: Bryan Ausinheiler, Caitlin Halferty, Toni Silver
Make-Up: SabrinaFosterMakeup.com

INJURY REHAB

with
RESISTANCE BANDS

CONTENTS

PART 1: OVERVIEW...................1

Introduction 2

History of Rehabilitative Exercises 4

Why Rehab with Resistance Bands? 6

Choosing a Band 8

The Rehabilitation Process...................... 10

FAQs 15

How to Use this Book............................. 18

PART 2: CORRECTIVE ROUTINES 21

Chronic Orthopedic Issues 22

Ankle/Foot 26

    Ankle/Foot Arthritis 28

    Sprained Ankle 30

    Achilles Tendon Issues...................... 31

Hip & Leg.. 33

    Hip Bursitis 35

    Arthritis of the Hip 37

    Groin Strain 38

    Iliotibial Band Fasciitis 39

Knee 41

    Bursitis of the Knee Joint 43

    Knee Ligament Injuries...................... 44

    Meniscus Injuries 46

    Arthritis of the Knee 47

Lower Back Region 49

Neck 51

Hands & Wrists.................................... 53

    Arthritis of the Hands & Wrist 55

    Carpal Tunnel Syndrome..................... 57

Elbow 58

Shoulder.. 60

Tendinitis & Bursitis.............................. 64

Shoulder Impingement 66

Arthritis of the Shoulder Joint 67

Rotator Cuff Injuries 68

PART 3: EXERCISES 69

Shoulder Series

    Pull-Down 70

    Lat Pull-Down 71

    Reverse Fly 72

    Frontal Raise 73

    Lateral Raise 74

    Sword Fighter 75

    Downward Sword Fighter 76

    Shrug....................................... 77

    Band Push-Up 78

    Horizontal Chest Press 79

    Incline Chest Press......................... 80

    Fly 81

    Chest Fly 82

    Shoulder Press 83

    Rotator Cuff—Internal Rotation 84

    Rotator Cuff—External Rotation............ 85

Back & Torso Series

    Long Row 86

    Torso Curl 87

    Chair Sit-Up 88

    Pelvic Lift 89

    Reverse Wood Chop......................... 90

    Side Bend 91

    Torso Rotation 92

    Archery Pull................................ 93

Arm & Hand Series

    Biceps Curl 94

    Reverse Curl 95

    Horizontal Triceps Extension 96

    Triceps Extension 97

    Forearm Flexion & Extension 98

    Wrist Fold 100

    Racehorse 101

    Squeezer 102

Leg & Hip Series

    Gas Pedal 103

    Seated Leg Press 104

    Leg Curl 105

    Squat 106

    Squat Shuffle 107

    Forward Lunge 108

    Side Lunge 109

    Leg Abduction & Adduction 110

    Reverse Leg Extension 111

Corrective Stretches

    Neck Rotation 112

    Tennis Watcher 112

    Soup Can 113

    Elbow Touch 114

    Shoulder Box 115

    Shoulder Roll 115

    Over the Top 116

    Choker 116

    Picture Frame 117

    Mad Cat 117

Long Body Stretch 118

Side Bend 118

Single Knee to Chest 119

Piriformis Stretch 120

Figure 4 120

Quad Stretch 121

Straight-Leg Stretch 122

Inner Thigh Stretch 122

Iliotibial Band Stretch 123

The Butterfly 123

Pretzel 124

Standing Hip Flexor 125

Rear Calf Stretch 125

Drop-Off Stretch 126

Rear Calf Stretch with Strap 126

Gas Pedal Stretch 127

Heel Raise/Heel Drop 127

Ankle Circle 128

Self-ROM 128

Ankle Roller 129

Finger Spreader 129

Finger Tap 130

V-W Stretch 131

Seated Wrist Stretch 132

Standing Wrist Stretch 132

Inward/Outward Wrist Move 133

Index 134

Acknowledgments 137

About the Author 138

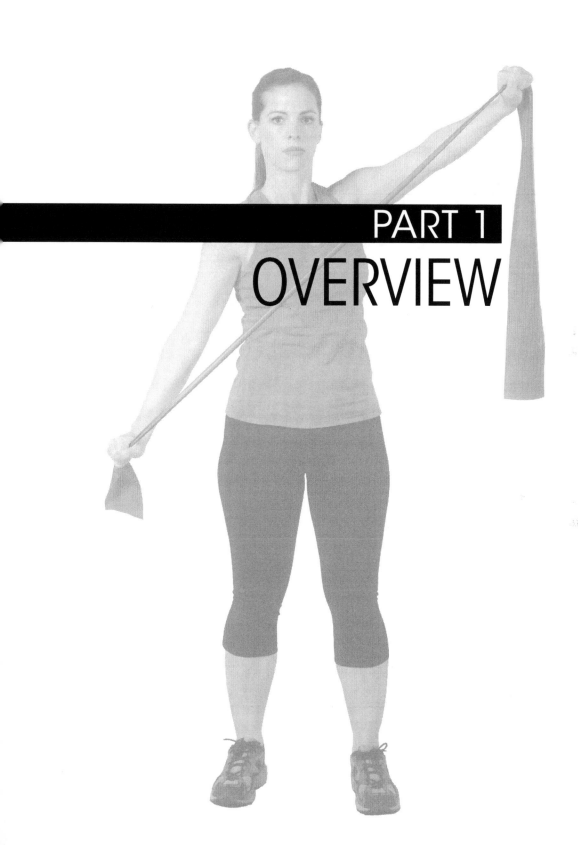

PART 1
OVERVIEW

INTRODUCTION

The world of health and fitness is a complex one. Since lack of exercise contributes to diabetes, high blood pressure and other assorted sedentary health concerns, we're told to exercise, but too much exercise causes overstress and injury to our joints and muscles. Additionally, while exercise can make us feel high, too much can bring us pain and soreness.

The answer is to train smart. When you hurt, know when to back off and use corrective exercises. Today, doctors understand the importance of both passive therapies and rehabilitative exercise. While medical science continues to make great advances in surgical and pharmacologic treatments, exercise physiologists are also proving that simple interventions such as proper body mechanics and corrective exercise can play a significant role in decreasing the incidence and severity of arthritis and orthopedic injuries.

One of the goals of rehabilitation today is functional fitness, in which the expected outcome is to maximize the potential for full return of pre-injury status and minimize the chance of re-injury. Just having big arm muscles doesn't mean you're able to throw a ball long and hard. Functional fitness means being fit for your desired activities.

Exercise bands are marvelous corrective-exercise tools with which to rehab a condition. They're also inexpensive, portable and very adaptable, available in a range of intensities. Almost any condition can benefit from using resistance bands—it's not uncommon to see physical therapists engage clients in the usage of bands. Even major-league pitchers have an assortment of bands hanging in the bullpen to be used for warm-up.

In this book you'll find basic information about many common conditions and some corrective exercises that are often used in a rehab setting. While this book is not intended to replace medical advice, I hope that your health provider will use it as a guide to help you facilitate your recovery. The philosophy of this book is that knowledge is power, and the more you know about your condition, the more you'll be an equal partner in your health care. Not every exercise in this book is perfect for everyone. However, these exercises have stood the test of time and are considered evidence-based exercises. If you choose to start performing the exercises in this book without medical input, start slowly and monitor how you feel. If you feel worse two hours post-exercise, back off and don't mask pain with overuse of medications.

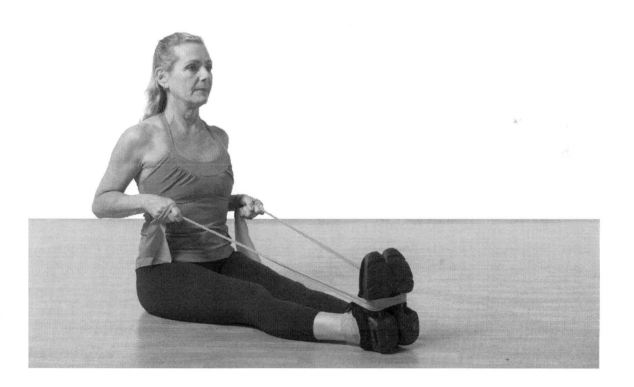

HISTORY OF REHABILITATIVE EXERCISES

Prior to World War II, a physical therapy prescription was often considered complete when all it mentioned was heat, rest and massage. Rehabilitation meant little more than passive rest and range-of-motion exercises facilitated by the therapist. Old-school rehab often just "worked" on the injured part of the body and neglected the others. If exercise was even prescribed it was only listed vaguely.

However, during World War II a revolution of sorts occurred in the field of physical medicine, and therapeutic exercise began to gain acceptance. Physicians began to increasingly become aware of the role that corrective exercise could play in fully restoring soldiers to complete function.

In the 1970s, Dr. Ken Cooper and other exercise physiologists showed how proper regular exercise can be both a preventive tool for better health and a rehabilitation tool for improved function. Today, rehabilitation is not about rest but rather active rehabilitation that integrates both passive and active measures.

Current research continues to show that regular prudent physical activity when preformed in a consistent manner is both healthful and beneficial to quality and quantity of life. In simple terms, if it's physical, it's therapeutic! Many of the protocols learned from the field of sports medicine to prepare elite athletes for competition and to return them to the playing field are now available to all of us. The current concept in therapy is to involve a total restoration of the system, which is sometimes called a "mind-body" approach.

WHY REHAB WITH RESISTANCE BANDS?

To improve strength, all you need to do is apply resistance to the muscle. As the muscle adapts to that load, challenge it again with more resistance. Thus, the proper term for strength training is "progressive load." There's an old myth in which a Greek god started lifting a baby cow every day; as the cow grew in size and weight, his muscles adapted to the load and he developed great amounts of strength. Today, we don't need to lift a cow to improve strength. We have a variety of equipment available to do so, including barbells, dumbbells, machines, exercise bands and even our own body weight.

For the purpose of therapy, however, resistance bands are often preferred. They're the perfect tool for rehab since they're light, easy to adjust and add resistance in multiple directions. Their adaptability and versatility also make them suitable for all levels. Additionally, resistance bands are not only inexpensive, they're very portable and can be carried and used anywhere. A set of exercise bands that ranges in intensity from super easy to extremely hard can fit in a small bag.

Initially surgical tubing was the material used for rehabilitation purposes. In the mid-1970s when I was a therapist on a spinal cord unit, we'd borrow various-sized surgical tubing from the warehouse and attach it to a bed frame as a means to foster improved strength for those individuals who were too weak to even lift a 2-pound weight. Today, resistance bands of all sizes and colors have replaced the brown surgical tubing we stole from the medical supply shed.

Almost any exercise that can be done with a piece of exercise equipment can be done with an exercise band. I personally think even more adaptations exist with band training than with weights or machines. The bands come in varying resistances so, as you get stronger, you can purchase heavier resistance bands in order to accommodate your improvements in strength. In addition, you're less likely to re-injure yourself with a resistance band, and load progression can be done slowly.

CHOOSING A BAND

Resistance bands are typically made of latex and come in several shapes and intensities. They're commercially available at most sporting-goods stores and therapy outlets and through online vendors. Selecting the correct band for your goals and body type is critical for obtaining ideal results. Some bands are designed to be grasped anywhere, while others come with handles, straps that can be wrapped around your legs or ankles and attachments that secure the band to the door.

Depending on the manufacturer, the color of the band generally denotes the intensity. Usually a light color such as pink and yellow is the easiest resistance, green and red moderate and dark gray and black very intense. However, please keep in mind that no standards exist between band manufacturers (one manufacturer's pink band may be much harder than another manufacturer's pink band), so select the band you use based on

how it feels rather than the color. There are basically two forms of resistance bands: flat and tubular.

Flat bands: These are the most common type of exercise band used. They're inexpensive and available latex-free for those with a latex allergy. Sometimes these bands come in rolls and can be cut for specific purposes; they can also be purchased pre-cut. Most exercises can be completed with a 3- to 6-foot piece of band; you can "choke up" on the band to make it fit your needs. You may also purchase handles specially made for them, although I've found that just wrapping flat band around a small piece of PVC pipe provides a wonderful handle. Even better, PVC pipe can be purchased in a variety of diameters to fit arthritic hands.

If you've never used bands before, start with the flat band and progress from there. This type of band is generally what clients are

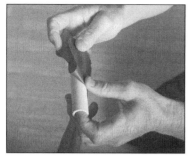
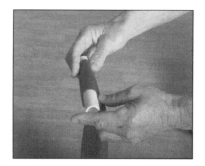
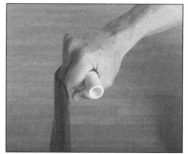

Band wrapped around PVC pipe

given for "home programs" when they've completed physical therapy.

Tubular bands: These are more durable than the flat kind and come with padded handles. You may even find tubing with adjustable handles in order to adapt the length of the tubing to the individual; however, most are available only in a pre-cut length. Nowadays exercise tubing comes in an array of options. Some resistance training bands are loops that can be wrapped around your limbs. You may also come across a figure eight-shaped band and a braided exercise tube.

In general, all the exercises in this book can be done with either type of band. Most of my students have found that the flat band works very well for performing corrective exercises as well as for general conditioning. Some have two or three bands depending on the body part being exercised.

USING BANDS SAFELY

While resistance band training is considered safe, there are some things you should keep in mind for best results. Regardless of the type of band you use, know that it will deteriorate over time due to exposure to the elements and oil from your hands. Therefore, make sure to check it before you use it; minor cracks will cause it to snap and possibly slap you in the face. An overly worn band also loses its ability to provide adequate resistance, so replace it frequently. One way to lengthen its lifespan is to store it in a plastic bag with baby powder and keep it out of direct sunlight. If you're using attachments, make sure they're securely fastened.

Here are other points to consider when using resistance bands:

- Incorrect placement of your hands on the band can allow you to cheat and could set you up for an injury.

- Remember to control the band—don't let it control you! Allowing the band to recoil compromises the quality of the training session.

- Since the resistance changes with the angle and speed of the movement, it's difficult to quantify the level of the resistance. Listen to your body and work to the level of fatigue that feels correct for you.

THE REHABILITATION PROCESS

Rehabilitation from an injury or dysfunction is often a long and frustrating process. A former chief of orthopedics surgery once told me that we can do remarkable things but we can never make the body better than the original equipment you were born with.

His advice was to take care of your joints—you want them to last a lifetime. If you push too fast and hard, you only re-injure yourself. This concept is very relevant when it comes to our joint health. Happy joints equal a happy life. So if you're injured, be proactive about performing corrective exercises as early as possible.

The desired goal of a corrective exercise program is to match the correct prescription of exercise to the person's condition. This is not to suggest that exercise is some type of magic bullet, nor to infer that exercise in and of itself can take the place of medicine. However, corrective exercise can play an irreplaceable role in the process of returning folks to their pre-injury status. The tricky part is to match the program to the person's unique characteristics.

Unfortunately, many people lack access to a physician with special training in physical medicine and are often left to implement a corrective exercise program by themselves. Other times, people turn to a personal trainer who often doesn't have specialized training and uses a one-size-fits all approach. The ideal situation is to have a partnership with a physical therapist who can design a home-based program that you can perform on your own.

PROFESSIONAL THERAPY

Before starting any type of rehabilitation work, it's wise to have a health professional perform a complete evaluation of you. She'll often compare both active and passive range of motion, as well as any deficits in strength, and compare the affected side to the non-affected side. After the evaluation, she may determine what stage you're currently at and base your corrective exercises on your status.

Your health professional will guide you along the steps, with your pain level and range of motion being key criteria for how much you should or shouldn't do. It's important to keep in mind that each person has his or her own timetable for recovery, and that the absence of pain is not a sign to return to "normal" activity. Also, many times people develop compensatory adjustments to make up for functional deficits, which may lead to further dysfunction. Justifying compensatory movements is generally not acceptable as these movements might only cause trauma further up or down the kinetic chain.

The rehabilitation goals occur in three stages: acute, recovery and functional. If you're undergoing surgery, an extra stage (pre-habilatation) might be suggested.

PHASE 1—ACUTE PHASE

The acute phase focuses on preventing further harm, decreasing the signs and symptoms of injury and hastening the healing process. A trained therapist should oversee this phase of rehabilitation. A combination of NSAIDs, rest, ice and heat may be suggested.

PHASE 2—RECOVERY PHASE

The goal of the recovery phase is to prevent further injury and pain using the methods discussed above. The corrective exercise program will focus on regaining body strength, muscular balance and stability of the joint. The corrective exercise routine may aim to foster functional range of motion and improve neuromuscular control and coordination.

PREHABILITATION

Prehabilitation is a relatively new concept in which you meet with your health professional and discuss any areas you should work on prior to a surgery. She might suggest you strengthen your arms so that you can use a walker easier after a hip replacement, or she may show you gentle gait and balance exercises to strengthen your quads so you can function better after knee surgery. Prehabilitation can be any form of exercise that will hasten your recovery after a procedure, be it corrective exercise to improve range of motion or strength training. Occasionally, prehab exercises are so effective that a person might end up not needing the procedure at all.

TOP TIPS FOR CORRECTIVE TRAINING

The following tips will help you gain the most from your program.

1. Make sure you're cleared by your health professional to engage in resistance band training. Don't make pain!

2. Always prepare your body for training by performing a few warm-up moves, taking a warm shower, and/or dressing in layers to keep your area of concern warm and supple.

3. Always execute the movement at a controlled speed with proper posture and with sound biomechanics. Quality reps over quantity of reps are best.

4. Never hold your breath. Holding your breath can increase your blood pressure. Instead, exhale on the hardest part of the exercise and inhale on the return portion.

5. Listen to your body. If you have pain, stop. If you have pain 2 hours post-exercise, re-evaluate the exercise and the intensity of the band.

6. Be regular. Ideally aim to perform some form of training several times a week. If you don't feel any strain, try increasing to more times per week. More intensity is not needed in corrective exercise.

7. Perform the exercise through the full range of motion.

8. Train, don't strain. It's okay to back off, but don't quit.

9. Consider performing some gentle active stretches or icing your joint after your routine if it's allowed by your health provider.

10. Be pro-active about your health. Take care of yourself so you can take care of others.

11. Greatness lies not in being strong, but in the correct use of strength.

12. When performing corrective exercises, be in the moment. You need to control the band—don't let the band control you.

13. Make this time "me" time, a mind-body experience.

PHASE 3—FUNCTIONAL PHASE

The functional phase can be done with an adaptive fitness personal trainer or by yourself—as long as you/he/she stays within the scope of practice and is following the protocols set forth by the medical professional. Once you've regained full functional recovery, evaluate the circumstances that may have caused your condition and adapt your lifestyle and behaviors. At this stage, learn exercises that foster improved stabilization of joints, practice proper posture, improve multi-plane range of motion and correct any strength irregularities. Sport-specific drills and functional activities of daily living should be included.

PRACTICE PERFECT POSTURE

Most people know that poor posture can lead to back pain, but posture also plays an important role in overall health. For instance, the rounded-shoulder, forward-head posture (think turtle) is often seen in people who swim a lot using the crawl/freestyle stroke without strengthening the opposing muscle group and stretching the chest muscles. This decreased flexibility of the chest and shoulder can set the stage for shoulder problems. Another example is limping on a simple sprained ankle; this can adversely affect your body mechanics and throw your hip off.

Experts now understand that if one body part is misaligned, overused or hurt, it can affect the mechanics somewhere along the kinetic chain. Look for the image of good posture above. Notice that the ear, shoulder, hip and ankle are all on the same vertical line. Any deviation from this alignment can lead to a multitude of issues, from neck and shoulder problems to lower back pain. Of course, plenty of things, like working a desk job, sitting in a cramped airplane seat, and fixing a car will challenge your ability to maintain good posture. That's why you should assess your posture several times a day.

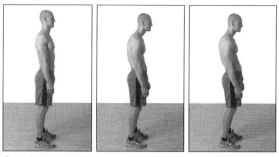

Good posture (left); poor posture (center, right)

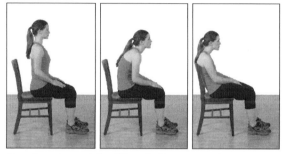

Good posture while sitting (left); poor posture (center, right)

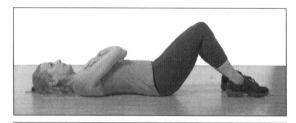

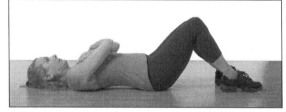

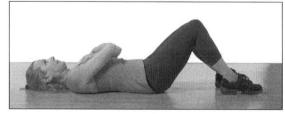

Proper neutral spine (top); lower back too arched (middle); lower back too flat (bottom)

The easiest way to do this is to stand with your back against a wall, with your heels no more than 6 inches from the wall. Place your bottom to the wall then attempt to place your upper back and the base of your head to the wall, keeping your chin down. If you have very compromised posture, start with just placing your bottom against the wall; as you improve, take your time trying to get your upper back against the wall before finally attempting to get your head to the wall. Some older people with severely compromised posture never get their head to the wall, so start today before it's too late. Practicing proper posture will reduce issues in all parts of the body, from head to toe.

Take a moment and honestly appraise your posture by looking in the mirror.

POSTURE CHECK

Before embarking on a corrective therapy routine, take a moment to practice proper standing posture.

1. Stand with your weight evenly distributed over the balls of your feet and heels.

2. Tuck your tailbone between your legs until you feel balanced. Imagine your pelvis as a bucket of water and you don't want any to spill.

3. Make the distance from your belly button and your chest as far apart as possible, and gently draw your bellybutton in and then place an imaginary apple under your chin. From a front view, you have a straight line down from your chin through the middle of your chest and pelvis falling midway between your spread feet. From a side view, your ears, shoulders and hips should be aligned (page 13). A mental picture that works for my students is to think of your body as a tube of toothpaste, with all the forces squeezing you in and upright. When sitting, keep your ears aligned over your shoulders and your shoulders aligned over your hips; your knees are aligned over your ankles.

FAQS

Below are frequently asked questions about starting a corrective exercise program.

Q. How much resistance should I start with?

A. Start easy and gradually increase the number of repetitions (reps) until you can do 3 to 5. Using resistance that's too light won't make improvements, while resistance that's too heavy may cause injury. Slowly progress, adding 1 to 2 reps each week. When you can do 10 to 12 reps with no pain, consider increasing to 2 sets. Once you reach this level, consider slowly increasing the reps to 15. When you can do 1 set of 15 without any undue discomfort, try a second set, starting with 5 reps and working up to 2 sets of 15 reps. Once you can perform 2 sets of 15 reps, it's time to upgrade to a stronger band and repeat the protocol all over again. Remember: The phrase "no pain, no gain" is insane.

Q. How many sets do I need to perform?

A. Start out with one set for a few weeks then slowly progress to two sets for an additional few weeks. You may increase to three sets. Keep in mind that quality reps and sets is more important than mindless reps, and that proper form is the key to beneficial corrective exercise. If you feel more pain 2 hours post-exercise, consider backing off the next time and maybe consider the application of heat/cold and massage. When you first start out, only do your exercises every other day. Once your body becomes accustomed to the work, you may be able to perform your rehab exercises daily, just like brushing your teeth. Slow and steady wins the corrective exercise race.

Q. Do I need to rest between sets?

A. Allowing the muscles to recover is a good idea. Shorter rest will improve muscular endurance, but you may want to rest longer (1 to 3 minutes) if you're using heavy resistance. Consider applying ice after a session if instructed to by your therapist. Some therapists may want you to apply heat in the form of a shower or heat pack before you exercise.

Q. Should I strength train daily?

A. It depends. If you train hard and heavy, the muscles worked need approximately 48 hours to replenish their energy (glycogen stores) and increase protein synthesis, which assists in growth of the muscle as long as adequate nutrition is provided. Allowing adequate recovery reduces the incidence of injury. However, since your corrective resistance band training is generally not strenuous, it may be ok for you to exercise daily. Just pay attention to how your body responds afterward.

Q. Does the order I train in matter?

A. Generally, it's best to train large muscles such as legs, chest and back first. Also, it's suggested to do compound exercises (such as the chest press) prior to isolated-muscle exercises (such as arm curls). If you're doing a total-body workout, make sure you do your corrective exercises early in the routine so that they're not neglected.

Q. How long do I follow my routine?

A. The human body is very efficient so it adapts to a challenge rather quickly. Changing your routine by increasing the load or reps or inserting new exercises periodically is wise.

Q. Is corrective resistance band training dangerous for me if I have high blood pressure or heart issues?

A. Strenuous strength training can cause a sudden spike in blood pressure. If you have high blood pressure or any cardiovascular concerns, speak with your health professional about the best training intensity for you. If you have any cardiovascular issues, keep the following suggestions in mind:

- Avoid holding your breath—breathe easily and continuously.

- Lift lighter—do more reps instead of going heavy.

- If you experience dizziness or chest pain, STOP!

Q. How do I prepare for a corrective exercise program?

A. Include a thermal warm-up to prepare your body for exercise. This could be light, aerobic activity that limbers up the muscles you plan to engage, or a warm shower or heating pad on the area that requires corrective exercise.

Q. Do I need to stretch?

A. After your corrective workout, it's recommended that you spend 5 to 15 minutes stretching the muscles you engaged in your workout. Then finish up with some icing of the affected areas, if approved by your health professional.

TEN TIPS FOR HEALTHY JOINTS

The areas that are most at risk of injury are the neck, the lower back, the knees and the shoulders. Here are a few ways to keep them healthy.

1. Identify a problem early to keep it small. Anytime you sense that you're having a joint issue, an early appointment with your health professional will hasten your recovery. Playing with pain will only increase the risk of a minor issue becoming a major issue.

2. Avoid overtraining. Maintain a sensible balance between training and proper rest.

3. Balance the volume and intensity of your training.

4. Know your safe and pain-free range of motion.

5. Avoid high-risk exercises/activities such as squats, dead lifts, presses behind the neck, and most CrossFit activities.

6. Train, don't strain. Cross-train to prevent overuse syndrome.

7. Include exercises to condition the supporting muscles of the joint.

8. Train smart—poor form and execution equals injury. Any abuse of your body today may haunt you later in life.

9. Understand the proper mix of reps and sets for maximum gain and minimum risk.

10. Learn how to prepare for activity, whether it be pre-season conditioning or pre-game joint readiness.

HOW TO USE THIS BOOK

This is the type of book you'll refer to over and over again. You may need to only read the section on shoulder exercises this time if you have a rotator cuff injury. However, next year, after you've completed training for a half-marathon, the knee and hip section might be useful.

A famous sports medicine doctor I know gives some of my other books to his patients, and he circles the exercises that are best for them at the present time. Then, at the next visit, he adds different exercises to his patient's corrective rehab program. Your health provider could do the same for you. This book was never intended to diagnose a condition or to replace your therapist; consider this a supplement to your physical therapy consultations. If you choose to start performing the exercises in this book without medical input, start slowly and monitor how you feel. If you feel worse 2 hours post-exercise, back off and don't mask pain with overuse of medications.

DESIGNING YOUR CORRECTIVE EXERCISE PROGRAM

This book can be used many ways. You can use it in concert with the treatment plan your health professional has set up for you, or you can follow the pre-set programs in Part 2. You can even be creative and design your own routine.

As you design your corrective resistance-training program, make every effort to make it fun and functional. Since we tend to repeat those things that we enjoy and avoid things that are boring, make your program enjoyable.

To gain the most return on investment from your corrective fitness routine, it's critical that you understand the concept of dose and response. Too much "dose" causes a bad response, such as discomfort and re-injury, while too little dose causes no response and thus no benefits. A regular "dose" of 15 to 20 minutes may be all you need to regain your former form and function. If you're too busy to commit to that amount of time, then you must be too busy to keep returning for follow-up doctor's visits. Ask yourself, if not now, when? Unfortunately, next year may be too late. Perhaps that little problem today may become a chronic disability later.

TRACKING YOUR PROGRESS

I've included blank charts in order to allow you to create your own individualized routine. Feel free to make copies of them. Make your routine a living document that you adapt and modify as you progress or sometimes even regress, changing sets, reps and exercises as you feel your body needs. Always keep in mind that you're the captain of your body and that one person's medicine is another person's poison. Your program should be special to you.

When designing your corrective exercise program, consider the following:

1. Understand how any of your pre-existing medical conditions interplay with your current orthopedic issues. Always solicit input about indications and contraindications from your health professional.

2. Train smart, not hard! Remember the 2-hour rule: Don't make pain! If you feel worse after a session, back off.

3. Match the activity to your personality. Remember that exercise does not need to be strenuous to be healthful. A sound exercise program can be the proactive means to prevent a problem as well as to recover from a problem.

4. Listen to YOUR body and heed what it says. This means select one or two exercises that you think matches your pain tolerance and skill set. Start with 3 to 5 reps and perform them very slowly, staying mindful of how you feel while doing them and afterward. If you feel worse, back off and try one or two other exercises.

5. Keep the FUN in the FUNdamentals of your program, otherwise you won't do it. It's better to do a little bit of anything than a lot of nothing. Make corrective exercise time a priority. These exercises can be done anywhere so no excuses.

Does your hip pain limit your recreational activities? Know that what happens above or below the affected area plays a significant role in fixing the problem. Too often a person who spends too much time strengthening one area and neglecting the opposing muscle group may get more inflexible, thereby compounding problems. However, too much stretching can compromise the stability of a joint. Overly lax joints can be just as bad as overly tight muscles. Think balance and symmetry.

DOING IT RIGHT

Everyone knows that physical activity and exercise are good for the human body. Unfortunately, in our zest to get fit, we often hurt ourselves because we're using outdated principles or being convinced by some faulty assumptions. Some exercises have been around so long that it seems irreverent to question their efficacy. Often training methods get adopted and later institutionalized based on anecdotal information rather than science. Good sense suggests that even proper exercise, if done correctly, can be injurious to your health.

One biomechanics expert stated that at least 90 percent of exercise programs include some exercises that are as detrimental as they are valuable. The key when determining if an exercise is correct is: Does it pass the benefits-to-risk ratio quiz?

Please take a few moments every so often to re-evaluate your fitness program. Doing so regularly may help prevent future injuries and also explain why you're hurting.

- Am I doing this exercise/activity correctly, the way I was instructed?

- Do I know the benefits of this exercise/activity?

- Do I know if there are any risks associated with this exercise/activity?

- Do I feel ok while doing this exercise/activity?

- Do I feel better after doing this exercise/activity?

- Do I feel worse after doing this exercise/activity?

- Could I receive the same benefits doing a different exercise/activity?

- Am I masking my pain with medication so that I can do the exercise?

If your trainer fails to be mindful of the above considerations, find a different trainer. Any exercise that has made it into your routine should provide maximum return on investment.

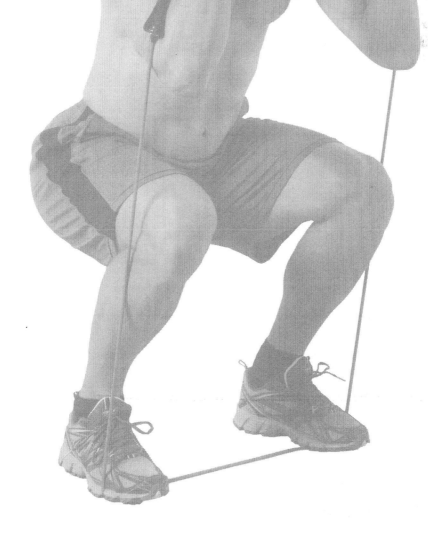

PART 2
CORRECTIVE ROUTINES

CHRONIC ORTHOPEDIC ISSUES

Many of our chronic orthopedic problems come from the abuse and misuse of our muscles and joints. As a result, we've disturbed the delicate balance of our muscular-skeletal system. Since our bodies are designed to move, we often don't feel the pain and manifestations of those misuses and abuses.

While no one wants to get old, getting older is impossible to avoid. As the sands of time pass, our physiological systems change. Our lean muscle mass, bone mass and coordination decrease, our ligaments and tendons lose elasticity, and our reaction time diminishes. Proper nutrition and lifestyle can prolong the advent of these outcomes but they do eventually occur in most people.

Therefore, to recover from an injury or to prevent one, we need to create a better-balanced body. Even the best physical therapy in the world won't help if you continue to habitually engage in poor body mechanics and misuse your body.

A number of sports medicine experts believe that several factors play a role in the development of orthopedic problems:

- Muscle imbalances
- Asymmetrical issues of gait and leg length
- Poor posture/body mechanics
- Improper muscle recruitment
- Trauma/injury

- Misuse and abuse (wear and tear)
- Not attending to minor injuries early
- Not understanding the delicate interplay of rest and training

Training smart, not hard, can lessen your likelihood of getting hurt or re-injured. Many sports medicine physicians believe that once you have an injury, your likelihood of re-injuring that area significantly increases. Just the absence of pain does not equate to being completely healed. Many of the conditions discussed in this section might've been prevented simply by understanding the following simple tips. What you do today can seriously affect your tomorrows.

- Train, don't strain—what you do today may contribute aches and pains in the future.
- Always perform your exercises with proper form.
- Don't neglect the small supporting (core) muscles of your joints. Most people focus on the superficial "show" muscles and forget the importance of these smaller but crucial muscles.
- Cross-train and utilize periodization. Don't overtrain the same muscles in the same manner, day in and day out.
- Exercise plays a major role in physical medicine when done in a prudent manner.

This section of the book addresses some of the more common conditions that manifest themselves as we engage in an active lifestyle and is designed to help you prevent problems with the use of resistance bands. If you pay attention to the variables discussed in this section, you may be the rare person who cruises through life without an acute or chronic problem. Train smart, not hard! Slow and steady wins the race!

If you already have an issue, you'll find post-rehabilitation exercises. Take time to rethink your motions and understand that your joints are not invincible. As one former professional athlete said later in life when he was limping around, "If I knew I was going to live this long, I would've taken better care of myself!" If you don't believe this, go to a professional sports team recognition game and see how those former athletes look. Too often they're walking with the help of canes or walkers.

COMMON ISSUES

The intent of this book is to provide basic information about common conditions that may occur and suggestions for maximizing your potential. While we may never be as good as we once were, we can still thrive with some adaptation to our lifestyle and activities. The goal of this book is to help you thrive, not just survive.

DISCLAIMER

"Corrective exercise" is a term for explaining the process of movements used to remediate a dysfunction. For corrective exercises to work, one must:

- Identify the problem (usually done by a health professional)

- Solve the problem (design a treatment plan)

- Engage in a dynamic corrective exercise routine, which changes as needed.

The corrective exercises in this section are designed to help you recover from an injury or maintain a healthy body part. Every effort was made to include only movements and exercises recognized by experts and therapists. If you're in the early stages of your rehabilitation, follow your medical professional's recommendations to the letter for the best results. The exercises they prescribe may or may not be in this book, and that's fine. An option is to take this book to your health professional and ask her to select those movements that best serve your condition. If you've fully recovered and have been discharged by your doctor, go ahead and select the exercises that appeal to you. As always, start slowly and perform them in a mindful manner, changing them up periodically.

GENERAL GUIDELINES FOR OSTEOARTHRITIS/DEGENERATIVE JOINT DISORDERS

Lack of physical activity is associated with muscle weakness, pain, joint stiffness, fatigue and decreased range of motion. Regular resistance training along with aerobic exercise (such as walking) and gentle range of motion has been shown to improve function and perhaps even reduce joint inflammation. Experts in the field of osteoarthritis suggest a regular program (2 to 3 times a week) of moderate-intensity strength training that addresses total body conditioning is helpful. Keeping your legs strong can reduce incidence of falls and improve mobility. Start slow and easy and evaluate your program regularly. If you feel more pain 2 hours post-exercise, consult your physician for guidance if need be.

Most experts recommend performing strength training with resistance bands. The Centers for Disease Control, along with the Arthritis Foundation, recommend the following to improve health and function:

1. Low-impact activities, such as water exercise, cycling and resistance training with bands

2. Resistance training 2 days a week and 2.5 hours of moderate aerobic exercise, which can be broken up into 10 to 30 minutes bouts as long as they don't increase pain or swelling

3. Water exercise (for more information, check out my water workout book, *Make the Pool Your Gym: No-Impact Water Workouts for Getting Fit, Building Strength and Rehabbing from Injury*)

Degenerative joint disease (DJD) is often called "wear-and-tear" arthritis because it's often caused by the misuse and abuse we put our bodies through. It's also called **arthritis or osteoarthritis** (OA), which is the inflammation and swelling of the cartilage and lining of a joint. The most common form of arthritis in the United States, osteoarthritis causes the cartilage to break down, commonly producing pain and stiffness. Osteoarthritis is often found in weight-bearing joints such as the ankle, hips and knees. It also occurs in the hands, lower back and any other joint. Arthritis is estimated to be a major crippler of Americans.

The causes of arthritis are multifactorial, including biomechanical issues as well as biochemical. Genetics, dietary issues, estrogen and bone density, along with joint looseness, obesity and lack of muscle, all contribute to arthritis. A physician should make the diagnosis of degenerative joint disease. The severity of degenerative joint disease ranges from mild to severe. In severe cases of degenerative joint disease, you may have an option of a joint replacement.

Once osteoarthritis has occurred, it's irreversible. Treatment focuses on maintaining function and decreasing pain. While osteoarthritis is seen in older adults, age alone is not a cause. Much of our joint discomfort is the result of how we've lived. That's why it's prudent to treat your joints kindly.

Sprains are a partial or complete tear of a ligament, which attach bone to bone. Ankle sprains, often the result of landing incorrectly and the joint moving in an abnormal direction, are reportedly the most common sports injury. If you incur a lateral sprain, you're at an increased risk of developing chronic instability of the ankle area. Sprains can be classified in different categories. A first-degree sprain is mild and involves minor stretching or tearing. A second-degree sprain is a bit more severe and involves the tearing of the ligament fibers; if this is accompanied by swelling and pain, seek medical attention. The severe, third-degree sprain is a complete tear, and frequently the person will hear a snap; surgery is often required.

Strains, commonly called "pulled muscles," are injuries involving the muscle-tendon connection. They're most often caused by using a muscle in a way that it's not trained for. Essentially, a strain is the overstretching or overstressing of a muscle. Strains have three classifications. A first-degree strain is mild and doesn't cause disability. A second-degree strain involves significant tearing of the fibers,

and recovery time can last several weeks. A severe, third-degree strain is the complete destruction of the muscle-tendon unit.

Tendinitis is the inflammation of a tendon, connective tissue that attaches a muscle to a bone. The most obvious example is perhaps the Achilles tendon (feel the back of your heel and follow it up to your calf muscle). As the muscle turns into a tendon it becomes more dense. The purpose of the tendon is to transmit force and help provide stability to the joint area. Tendinitis can be caused by irritation seen in overuse syndromes (think tennis elbow) or poor technique.

Bursitis is pain and swelling of the bursae, small fluid-filled sacs located in or near the joints. These sacs help cushion any tissues that rub against or slide over hard bone. Repetitive motions can result in bursitis, with elbows, hips and knees being commonly affected areas. Healing time varies due to the severity of the condition. Unfortunately, often many people never let the area heal fully before jumping back into the activity that caused the problem.

ANKLE & FOOT

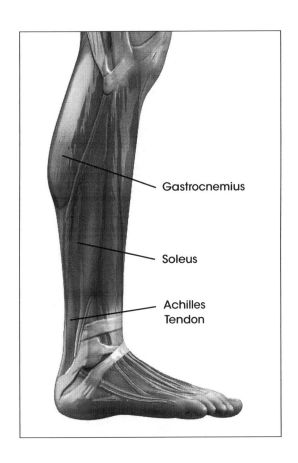

Gastrocnemius

Soleus

Achilles
Tendon

Many people have sprained ankles that require visits to the doctor. An ankle or foot problem is one of the fastest tickets to disability. How many times have we heard someone cry, "My feet are killing me"? The foot contains three main sections: the rear foot/heel, the midfoot and the forefoot. These three units must work together to allow for functional ambulation.

An elaborate network of muscles and ligaments holds the bones and joints of the foot and ankle together. The ankle joint is called upon to provide both stability for standing and mobility for ambulation. More and more research is finding that an issue in the foot/ankle can contribute to other problems up the kinetic chain, such as in the knee/hip/lower back. Just think how a stubbed toe throws your gait off and leads to other issues. Sometimes pain in the heel can even be referred pain from a spinal disc.

Here are some simple steps to prevent foot and ankle issues.

- Don't ignore foot pain.
- Select function over fashion when it comes to shoes.
- Stay lean—the heavier you are, the more force the ankle and foot need to absorb.
- Don't wear ankle weights.
- Protect your feet, whether doing water exercise or jogging.
- Consider cross-training, alternating between weight-bearing and non-weight-bearing activities.
- Replace running/active wear shoes every 500 miles. Running on shoes with worn-out soles contributes to injuries.
- Always running on the same side of the road can contribute to injuries due to the angle of the road.
- Have your feet measured each time you buy shoes to ascertain proper size.
- Wear your new shoes around the store for awhile before purchasing them.

ANKLE & FOOT ARTHRITIS

EXERCISES/STRETCHES	SETS	REP/TIME	REST
Lat Pull-Down *p. 71*			
Horizontal Chest Press *p. 79*			
Reverse Fly *p. 72*			
Frontal Raise *p. 73*			
Biceps Curl *p. 94*			
Seated Leg Press *p. 104*			
Gas Pedal *p. 103*			
Leg Curl *p. 105*			
Gas Pedal Stretch *p. 127*			
Tennis Watcher *p. 112*			
Straight-Leg Stretch *p. 122*			
Rear Calf Stretch *p. 125*			
Ankle Circle *p. 128*			
Shoulder Roll *p. 115*			
Finger Tap *p. 130*			

The foot and ankle area is very susceptible to arthritis due to the large number of joints required to handle a high level of load in this region. Combine this with some types of shoes people wear, from high heels to sandals with no support. If you have severe arthritis, you may need to rely on your upper body more to help you pull yourself up or to use a cane or walker to lessen the load on your lower extremities. Including exercises to improve upper-body strength would thus be a good idea, as would having a therapist teach you the proper use of a cane.

CAUSES

The causes of arthritis are varied. Some commonly believed causes of arthritis are:

— Wear and tear (misuse and abuse)

— Misaligned joints

— Excessive body weight

— Poor body mechanics

— Previous injury

TREATMENT OPTIONS

— Lifestyle modification and weight control

— Corrective exercise routines that include stretching and muscle strengthening

— Anti-inflammatory medication

— Injections

— Water exercise

— Active rest

— Gentle range of motion

— Applied ice or heat

— Ambulation aids such as canes, walkers or wheelchairs

— Surgery

— Patient education

— Re-evaluation of footwear

— Supportive devices

SPRAINED ANKLE

EXERCISES/STRETCHES	SETS	REP/TIME	REST
Gas Pedal *p. 103*			
Seated Leg Press *p. 104*			
Forward Lunge *p. 108*			
*Leg Abduction *p. 110*			
Leg Curl *p. 105*			
Side Lunge *p. 109*			
Self-ROM *p. 128*			
Ankle Circle *p. 128*			
Rear Calf Stretch *p. 125*			
Rear Calf Stretch with Strap *p. 126*			
Gas Pedal Stretch *p. 127*			

Follow steps 1 and 2 only.

Being that we are two-footed creatures, our ankles are called upon to perform remarkable activities. The most-reported injuries in the foot and ankle region are ankle sprains, with a sprain of the lateral ankle ligaments being the most common. A sprained ankle simply means that the ligaments are stretched beyond their normal limits. Sprained ankles run the gamut from mild to severe. If the pain is severe, consult your physician. If you have a sprained ankle, your goal is to restore strength and stability to the region. Do not perform any exercise until given approval by your physician.

CONTRIBUTING FACTORS

— Poor flexibility of the ankle

— Having an overly lax ankle joint

— Muscle weakness in the area

— Previous injuries to the area

TREATMENT OPTIONS

— Immobilization/brace

— Rest, Ice, Compression, Elevation (RICE)

— Decrease impact and load

— Seeing a physician or physical therapist

ACHILLES TENDON ISSUES

EXERCISES/STRETCHES	SETS	REP/TIME	REST
Gas Pedal p. 103			
Seated Leg Press p. 104			
Squat p. 106			
Squat Shuffle p. 107			
Forward Lunge p. 108			
Self-ROM p. 128			
Heel Raise/Heel Drop p. 127			
Ankle Circle p. 128			
Rear Calf Stretch p. 125			
Rear Calf Stretch with Strap p. 126			
Gas Pedal Stretch p. 127			

A very common sports-related condition, a tight Achilles tendon may cause pain that's located in your lower calf or along the back of your foot and above your heel, especially when stretching your ankle or standing on your toes. An abrupt stretching of the tendon when it's not properly conditioned or warmed up often causes tendon issues. For instance, a sprinter might get one at the start of a race. Men ages 30 and older are particularly prone to Achilles tendon injuries.

Many of these injuries are caused by tendinitis, in which the tendon becomes swollen and painful. In a severe Achilles tendon injury, too much force on the tendon can cause it to tear partially or rupture completely; with a full tear, you'll have difficulty flexing your foot or pointing your toes. An Achilles tendon injury can also result from flat feet, also known as fallen arches or overpronation. In this condition, the impact of a step causes the arch of the foot to collapse, stretching the muscles and tendons. Achilles tendon injuries are common in people who participate in ballistic sports such as running, gymnastics, dance, football, baseball/softball, basketball, tennis and volleyball.

Slow and steady is the way to treat this condition; approaching corrective exercises too quickly can worsen it. Do not do any exercise until given approval by your physician.

CAUSES

— Overuse

— Increasing physical activity too quickly

— Wearing high heels, which increases the stress on the tendon

— Foot problems

— Tight leg muscles or tendons

TREATMENT OPTIONS

— Follow your doctor's orders

— Evaluate your current exercise program

— Evaluate your footwear

— Switch to non-weight-bearing exercise programs

— Apply ice and heat as recommended by your doctor

— Engage in corrective exercises, such as stretching your calf muscles

HIP & LEG

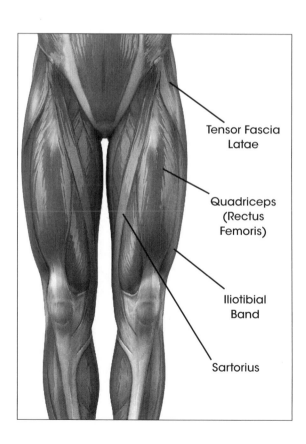

Tensor Fascia Latae

Quadriceps (Rectus Femoris)

Iliotibial Band

Sartorius

A ball-and-socket joint, the hip joint is often called the workhorse of the joints. It's stable due to the deep set of the neck of the femur resting inside the pelvis. This design allows the leg to move in various directions while being able to withstand heavy loads.

Hip problems are a major concern for everyone, from young athletes to senior citizens. Anytime you sit to stand, jump, run, bike or swim, your hip joint is activated. Due to its design, the hip joint allows for numerous motions, such as:

- Flexion (bringing the leg forward)
- Extension (taking the leg backward)
- Adduction (bringing the legs together)
- Abduction (taking the leg to the side)
- Circumduction (drawing circles with the leg)
- Rotation (making circles with the hips)

Many factors can contribute to a hip problem. Two basic anatomical factors influence how well your hip performs. Some experts think that having a shallow acetabulum (socket) can set a person up for hip issues, as can inflexibility of the joint. Leg and foot issues, such as hobbling around after a broken foot or sprained ankle, can also contribute to hip dysfunction. Also, leg-length discrepancy can often disturb the functional relationships of the spine, pelvis, foot and long bones of the leg; this can result in hip and knee pain.

Experts believe that several major factors play a role in hip problems:

- Muscle imbalances of the hip
- Asymmetrical issues of gait and leg length
- Poor posture
- Improper muscle recruitment
- Trauma/injury
- Misuse and abuse (wear and tear)

For better hip health, stay mindful of these "hip hurters," which are common, high-risk exercises that can possibly contribute to a chronic issue later in life:

- Full leg presses or squats, where the thighs reach an angle that's less than 90 degrees
- Explosive plyometric moves
- Deep lunges that allow your knee to wobble or your knee to go past your toes (this can transfer excessive force to the hip and pelvic region)
- Running/jumping bleacher stairs (jumping down is especially traumatic for the hip joint)
- Poor biomechanics while cycling or running
- Rowing moves that compress the hip joint

The following addresses some of the most common hip conditions. This is by no means a comprehensive list, nor is the intent of this section to provide you a means of self-evaluation. Always consult with your primary care physician to determine what your specific issue is. The hip region can manifest pain from numerous sources other than the hip specifically. Hip pain can be referred from the lower back, for example.

HIP BURSITIS

EXERCISES/STRETCHES	SETS	REP/TIME	REST
Seated Leg Press p. 104			
Squat p. 106			
Squat Shuffle p. 107			
Forward Lunge p. 108			
Side Lunge p. 109			
*Leg Abduction p. 110			
Reverse Leg Extension p. 111			
Straight-Leg Stretch p. 122			
Inner Thigh Stretch p. 122			
Rear Calf Stretch p. 125			
Standing Hip Flexor p. 125			
Gas Pedal Stretch p. 127			

*Follow steps 1 and 2 only.

Technically called *trochanteric bursitis* (with the trochanter being the part of the femur that connects to the pelvis), the inflammation of the bursa sac of the hip region results in pain and/or discomfort. The most common causes of bursitis are injuries or damage to the bursa, which may trigger pain, swelling and redness in the location. Individuals with leg-length discrepancies are more predisposed to bursitis. In addition, chronic misuse of the joint will at some point result in an injury, especially if you're biomechanically predisposed to injury. If you have hip bursitis, do not perform conditioning exercises until cleared by your physician.

CAUSES

— Overuse, overtraining

— Misuse of the hip joint

— Lying on the hip(s) for long periods of time

— Infection

— Injury (falling on the hip)

— Improper posture while sitting or standing

- Any disease that affects the bones, such as arthritis
- Pedaling a bike that's not properly adjusted to your body
- Performing deep squats
- Running with improper support or always running on the same side of the street
- Performing high-impact activities

- Engaged in high-impact activities, such as jumping up and down from a box; many boot-camp moves can contribute to trauma to the lower extremities

TREATMENT OPTIONS

- Stop running or performing the contributing activity
- Have your leg length evaluated
- Have your "Q" angle evaluated
- Rest, ice, compression/support, elevation (RICE)

ARTHRITIS OF THE HIP

EXERCISES/STRETCHES	SETS	REP/TIME	REST
Gas Pedal p. 103			
*Seated Leg Press p. 104			
Squat (only to chair depth) p. 106			
Forward Lunge (only taking a small step) p. 108			
*Reverse Leg Extension p. 111			
*Leg Abduction p. 110			
**Straight-Leg Stretch p. 122			
Inner Thigh Stretch p. 122			
Rear Calf Stretch p. 125			

*within a small range of motion
**movement from the waist area only, do not force

The hip is the workhorse of the body and is commonly affected by osteoarthritis, a chronic and often crippling disease. Arthritis of the hip can be caused by many things, including birth defects of the joint, poor biomechanics in sports and at work, being overweight, and falls/injury.

While there is no cure to date, management options such as surgery, medications and corrective exercises exist. General exercise recommendations for people with arthritis of the hip include low-impact activities, gentle walking, water exercise and quick stop-and-go movements, one-leg stances, gentle stretching and cross-training.

GROIN STRAIN

EXERCISES/STRETCHES	SETS	REP/TIME	REST
Side Lunge (gentle) p. 109			
Leg Abduction & Adduction at Wall (gentle) p. 110			
Squat Shuffle p. 107			
Reverse Leg Extension p. 111			
Standing Hip Flexor p. 125			
The Butterfly p. 123			
Single Knee to Chest p. 119			

*Your routine is best determined by your therapist.

The common groin strain first appears as a minor issue. Perhaps you feel a sudden twinge of pain and/or weakness in the upper inside portion of the leg. The injury can include the following muscles: gracilis, pectineus, adductor group (brevis, longus, magus). These muscles are relatively small and minor players and are often neglected in conditioning programs. If not addressed early on, a groin strain can become a chronic issue that can take an inordinate amount of time to heal. It's often difficult to treat and can easily be aggravated even after you feel it has healed. In severe cases, there's internal bleeding. Do not perform conditioning exercises until you're cleared by your physician.

CAUSES

— Explosive movements (running, jumping)

— Muscle imbalances

— External leg rotation, such as when doing a cutting motion

TREATMENT OPTIONS

— Avoiding those muscles and using alternative means to stay fit; your doctor may suggest swimming, arm crank bikes or water walking

— Rest, ice, compression/support, elevation (RICE)

— Physical therapy

— Whirlpool treatments

— Water therapy

— Cryotherapy (ice massage)

— Ultrasound

— Wrapping

— Biomechanics evaluation

— Active rest

— Corrective exercises (strength/flexibility)

ILIOTIBIAL BAND FASCIITIS

EXERCISES/STRETCHES	SETS	REP/TIME	REST
Seated Leg Press p. 104			
Squat p. 106			
Forward Lunge p. 108			
Side Lunge p. 109			
Reverse Leg Extension p. 111			
Squat Shuffle p. 107			
Leg Abduction & Adduction p. 110			
Standing Hip Flexor p. 125			
Rear Calf Stretch p. 125			
Piriformis Stretch p. 120			
Single Knee to Chest p. 119			

The iliotibial (IT) band is a thick swath of fascia that runs from the outside of the pelvis, over the hip and along the outside of the knee, inserting just below the knee. One of its main jobs is to stabilize the knee during running. Manifesting itself as pain along the outside the thigh, iliotibial (IT) band fasciitis (sometimes called "iliotibial band syndrome") is the result of inflammation of the lower portion of the IT tendon. It's often caused by overuse, along with weakness in the muscular area above the kinetic chain, such as the leg abductor muscles. The band exercises suggested here address the strengthening of underused muscles such as the quadriceps (rectus femoris), glutes and iliopsoas.

CAUSES

— Trochantentic bursitis (page 35) causing pressure on the IT band

— Faulty biomechanics seen in poor running or cycling form

— Muscle imbalances

— Overuse

TREATMENT OPTIONS

— Anti-inflammatory medications

— Cryotherapy (ice massage)

— Electrical stimulation

— Corrective stretches

— Muscle re-patterning

— Taping

— Rest, ice, compression/support, elevation (RICE)

KNEE

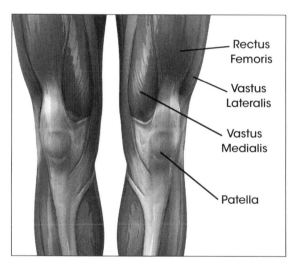

Rectus Femoris

Vastus Lateralis

Vastus Medialis

Patella

Imagine that every time you walk, jog, go up a step or worse yet, go down a step, the force on your knee is multiplied four times your body weight. If you are overweight or your quads are de-conditioned, the impact on your knee joint is further compounded. The bottom line is that if you have knee joint issues you should stay as lean as you can and keep your leg muscles as strong as you can without injuring the joint.

The knee joint is a convergence of the upper leg bone (femur), the fibula (one of the lower leg bones) and the patella (knee cap). Many muscles, such as the calf muscles, quadriceps and gluteal muscles, intersect in or around the knee joint. Overly tight leg muscles combined with lax muscles elsewhere may contribute to patella tendinopathy (jumper's knee) and iliotibial band syndrome.

The incidence of knee injuries is common, with approximately 80,000 to 100,000 anterior cruciate ligament (ACL) injuries occurring each year. Associated with poor body mechanics or muscle functions, many of the injuries don't involve contact and typically affect people ages 15 to 25. Many people with an ACL injury later go on to develop arthritis of the knee.

Very few injuries or diseases can cripple a person more than a bad knee. While modern surgical techniques have improved significantly over the past years, they're never as good as your original equipment. We need to do our best to keep our knee joint stable and strong. We now know that if we don't use our legs in a regular exercise pattern, the muscles will weaken through disuse syndrome. The weaker the quadriceps becomes the more difficult activities such as walking and climbing steps become. Causes of a knee problem can be an injury, overuse, engaging in outdated training techniques, muscle imbalances, a quick twist of the leg or just wear and tear (osteoarthritis) as we get older.

Knee pain is nature's way of telling you that something's wrong and you need to do something about it. Knee problems don't discriminate—they affect athletes and recreational hikers, as well as those with physically demanding jobs. Usually the best treatment for an aching knee is rest, along with either ice or heat and a gentle stretch. However, doing too much too soon only makes the muscles set the stage for a relapse. Also, too much rest contributes to weight gain, which also contributes to putting more strain on the new joint, so what's a person to do? Here are some recommendations:

- Stay as lean as possible—less excess weight means less load on the knee joint (every 1 pound of body weight translates to 4 pounds on the knee joint).

- Strengthen your quadriceps, hamstrings, adductors and abductors.

- Lengthen the gluteal muscles, IT band and calf muscles.

- If you're recovering from any problem, only do prescribed exercises.

- Even if you don't have any problems, start slowly and progress slowly.

- If you experience pain in the knee while exercising, back off and discuss it with your physician—avoid overtraining and activities such as full squats.

- When exercising, perform movements as biomechanically correct as possible. For example, not having proper leg extension when biking can cause trauma to the knee.

- Learn to use your knees in ways that will strengthen them, not strain them.

- When your knees hurt, rest them.

- Don't over use medicines to mask pain.

- If you have knock knees or are bowlegged, take special care to avoid strain and injury to the knee joint.

Remember: The goal of any exercise program pertaining to the knee joint is to improve strength, endurance and mobility. In addition, it takes strong leg muscles to have healthy knees.

BURSITIS OF THE KNEE JOINT

EXERCISES/STRETCHES	SETS	REP/TIME	REST
Seated Leg Press (halfway) *p. 104*			
Squat (quarter-way) *p. 106*			
Pelvic Lift *p. 89*			
Leg Curl *p. 105*			
Straight-Leg Stretch *p. 122*			
Standing Hip Flexor *p. 125*			

There are several bursa sacs within the knee area. Trauma and activities that apply too much direct pressure on the knee, such as kneeling, can cause bursitis. An inflamed bursa can result in the knee area swelling significantly, causing pain. This type of bursitis can be prevented by avoiding frequent kneeling or wearing knee pads when engaging in activities that might result in knee trauma. The suggested band exercises are aimed at regaining lost strength of the quadriceps.

TREATMENT OPTIONS

— In some cases the excess fluid may be aspirated

— Pain and anti-inflammatory medications

— Steroid injections

— Bracing, ice

— Avoiding direct pressure on knee

— Modification of exercise

KNEE LIGAMENT INJURIES

EXERCISES/STRETCHES	SETS	REP/TIME	REST
Pelvic Lift *p. 89*			
Side Lunge *p. 109*			
Squat Shuffle *p. 107*			
Seated Leg Press *p. 104*			
Forward Lunge *p. 108*			
Leg Curl *p. 105*			
Reverse Leg Extension *p. 111*			
Straight-Leg Stretch *p. 122*			
Standing Hip Flexor *p. 125*			
Rear Calf Stretch *p. 125*			

Knee injuries account for a majority of injuries seen in high school and college sports. Ligaments attach bone to bone to provide stability to a joint region. Recent studies indicate a relationship between neuro-muscle control and increased risk of ligament injuries, such as ACL injuries.

Knee ligament injuries can range from mild to severe and are often accompanied by intense pain and swelling. Since women have wider hips than men (this more-pronounced angle from the hip joint to the knee joint is commonly called the "Q" angle), they're more susceptible to knee issues. For instance, when females land after a jump, their knees turn inward, putting them at more risk in sports (such as soccer) that require landing and performing quick cuts.

The role of corrective exercise for knee ligament injuries is to provide a balanced strengthening program for the quadriceps and hamstrings, as well as the inner and outer thigh muscles. Also, try to learn to have the muscles fire in the proper order; a biomechanics expert can help here. Follow the advice of your attending medical personnel because they know the severity of your condition.

CAUSES

— Quick pivoting movements (such as when playing soccer or basketball)

— Quick deceleration

— Hyperextension

— Impact

TREATMENT OPTIONS

— Rest

— Pain medication

— Braces

— Physical therapy

— Surgery (when conservative treatments and physical therapy fail)

MENISCUS INJURIES

EXERCISES/STRETCHES	SETS	REP/TIME	REST
Pelvic Lift *p. 89*			
Seated Leg Press *p. 104*			
Leg Curl *p. 105*			
Side Lunge *p. 109*			
Leg Abduction & Adduction *p. 110*			
Squat *p. 106*			
Chair Sit-Up (halfway) *p. 88*			
Band Push-Up *p. 78*			
Straight-Leg Stretch *p. 122*			
Rear Calf Stretch *p. 125*			

The cartilage/cushion between the upper leg and the lower leg that functions to absorb some of the load you take with each step, the meniscus of the knee was once thought to be a useless remnant of the leg muscle. Today, experts understand that the meniscus has many functions, including joint stability and congruity.

The meniscus is often injured, although this is often the result of degenerative tears over time. The injury often occurs in people between 13 and 40 years of age as a result of falls or accidents. In older people, it's often caused by a quick turn or repeated stresses. Because the meniscus receives its blood supply by diffusion and has a low metabolic rate, healing is often slow. To prevent meniscus injuries, avoid trauma and hard falls to the knee region. As you get older, avoid quick pivots. Follow the advice of your attending medical personnel because they know the severity of your condition.

CAUSES

— Trauma, such as car accidents

— Falls, quick turns

TREATMENT OPTIONS

— Pain medication

— Immobilization of the joint

— Surgery

ARTHRITIS OF THE KNEE

EXERCISES/STRETCHES	SETS	REP/TIME	REST
*Seated Leg Press p. 104			
Squat (to chair quarter-way down) p. 106			
Forward Lunge p. 108			
Leg Curl (halfway or as tolerated) p. 105			
Gas Pedal p. 103			
Shrug p. 77			
Lateral Raises p. 74			
Horizontal Chest Press p. 79			
Archery Pull p. 93			
Long Row p. 86			
Triceps Extension p. 97			
Rear Calf Stretch p. 125			
Ankle Circle p. 128			
Straight-Leg Stretch p. 122			
Gas Pedal Stretch p. 127			

*within a safe range of motion with comfortable resistance

An estimated 46 million Americans have some form of arthritis. Arthritis is also the leading form of disability in Americans who are over 55 years old. There are many type of arthritis, but the most common form seen in the knee is the wear-and-tear form, commonly called osteoarthritis. This is the result of deterioration or loss of cartilage in the synovial joints. The strongest predictor of whether you'll get osteoarthritis is age, heredity, obesity and previous injury. The other type of arthritis is rheumatoid, which is a more systemic condition and should be given prescriptive exercises by a health professional.

Both types of arthritis can affect the knee. Symptoms include pain, stiffness, swelling and a grinding sensation in the joint due to the breakdown of the cartilage. Unfortunately, by the time you usually start feeling the effects of osteoarthritis of the knee, it's too late to be cured. Teaching young people to protect their knees goes a long way in minimizing the aches and pains of aging.

If you have osteoarthritis, your goal is to improve function, reduce muscle atrophy and foster greater joint mobility. Physical therapy, corrective exercises and water exercise are helpful with improving leg strength and maintaining a desirable weight. Upper-body exercises will keep your upper body strong in case you need a cane for assistance.

TREATMENT OPTIONS

— Physical therapy

— Corrective exercises

— Water exercise

— Moist heat and/or ice

— Medication

— Surgery

LOWER BACK REGION

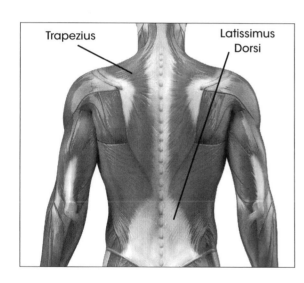

Trapezius

Latissimus Dorsi

The statistics regarding the number of Americans who experience lower back problems at some point in their lives are staggering. Each year Americans collectively spend billions of dollars treating lower back issues. Back pain is second only to the common cold for reasons to see a doctor and is the leading cause of absenteeism.

Due to the complex nature of the area, most likely because of the biomechanical dynamics between the spine and the pelvis, the lower back has potential for many issues. Some people may only complain of tightness or spasms, while others experience pain running down the back of their leg (called sciatica). The lower area of the spine takes most of the body's load when standing or sitting. That, combined with poor posture, tight hamstrings and weak abdominal muscles, sets the stage for chronic lower back problems. Many people are surprised to learn that their back issues can be resolved satisfactorily with proper body mechanics, corrective exercises and maintaining asymmetrical core strength (abdominal and lower back strength, hip and upper leg flexibility). If you can avoid being overweight, you can do a lot for your back.

There are many causes of lower back pain, from tumors and herniated discs to arthritis and muscle spasms. Since the cause is so varied, it's critical to see a medical doctor for proper diagnosis. Seek medical attention immediately if you're experiencing a leg pain or backache along with the following:

1. High fever

2. Loss of bowel and/or bladder function

3. Numbness or weakness in the legs or pelvic region

There are several common-sense tips you can heed to prevent lower back problems:

- When sitting, try to keep your knees higher than your hips.

- Learn proper biomechanics with regard to activities of daily living.

- Tone lax muscles (e.g., abdominal) and stretch tight muscles (e.g., hamstrings).

- Avoid twisting vigorously, such as when playing golf.

- Push rather than pull heavy loads.

- Avoid exercises that place a heavy load on the spine, such as old-fashioned sit-ups, straight leg lifts and military presses with weights.

- Engage in low-impact activities, such as water exercise and/or swimming.

TREATMENT OPTIONS

— Rest

— Ice or heat

— Medications such as non-steroid anti-inflammatories

— Electrical stimulation

— Physical therapy

— Corrective exercises

— Injections

— Acupuncture

— Massage therapy

EXERCISES/STRETCHES	SETS	REP/TIME	REST
Chair Sit-Up *p. 88*			
Torso Curl *p. 87*			
Side Bend *p. 118*			
Pelvic Lift *p. 89*			
Band Push-Up *p. 78*			
Single Knee to Chest *p. 119*			
Straight-Leg Stretch *p. 122*			
Mad Cat *p. 117*			

NECK

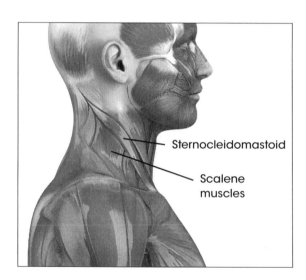

Sternocleidomastoid

Scalene muscles

A pain in the neck is truly a pain in the neck! "Neck pain" is an umbrella term that includes multiple symptoms and underlying causes. This type of pain can be the result of muscle-related issues such as spasms and stiffness, pinched nerves, an accident, arthritis, poor posture or sleeping incorrectly.

The neck is easily strained because of the way it's designed. It's basically a series of seven little blocks built atop each other in a manner that allows a significant amount of movement. The neck can move in almost every direction, and the muscles around the neck appear similar to a set of pulleys/levers and also serve as guide wires. Very often, a joint that has the potential to perform a large range of motion lacks stability. Neck problems can contribute to cervical tension syndrome, muscle tension headaches, facial pain and even shoulder and arm numbness. Sometimes neck issues can be the result of referred pain/numbness in the arm or upper back.

Upper back and neck issues increase with the degenerative process and can be accelerated by trauma and poor body mechanics. We've seen an increase in upper back and neck problems as more people have desk jobs that require sitting in a static position most of the day. The prolonged hunched-over position when typing places the neck and upper back in an unhealthy posture. Just getting up and looking left and right and up and down regularly could prevent many neck issues. In this section you'll notice exercises that improve flexibility and muscle tone of the supporting muscles of the upper back.

TREATMENT OPTIONS

— Rest with proper neutral posture

— Ice or heat

— Medications

— Physical therapy

— Corrective exercise

— Acupuncture

EXERCISES/STRETCHES	SETS	REP/TIME	REST
Sword Fighter *p. 75*			
Downward Sword Fighter *p. 76*			
Long Row *p. 86*			
Shrug *p. 77*			
Reverse Fly *p. 72*			
Archery Pull *p. 93*			
Mad Cat *p. 117*			
Tennis Watcher *p. 112*			
Long Body Stretch *p. 118*			

HANDS & WRISTS

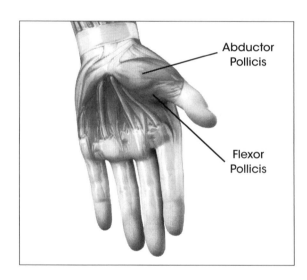

Abductor
Pollicis

Flexor
Pollicis

In today's world of electronic notepads and cell phones, our wrists and hands take on a lot of use, resulting in chronic overuse. Until your wrists start to be painful or get stiff, you may not realize how much you depend on your hands, fingers and wrist. They all appear to work as a unit.

The wrist can be strained, sprained or broken, and is frequently injured, either by falling on it with an outstretched arm or simply overusing it. Without a fully functioning wrist, our hand motions are limited. As we all know, the hands include the fingers and thumbs. Without a properly functioning thumb, our precise motions would be limited.

Many of the problems that are seen in the wrist, hands and fingers can be prevented with proper biomechanics, body awareness, taking regular breaks, performing corrective hand exercises, and having properly designed workstations and tools. Engaging in corrective exercises that build strength and improve functional range of motion should be a part of everyone's daily routine. Prevention and early detection can go a long way in protecting your wrist joint.

Taping and/or bracing the fingers or wrist is a good way to return to your activity. In addition, using the resistance band to do wrist curls is a good way to keep your forearm conditioned. Some occupational therapists will even ask their patients to place a rubber band around their fingers and spread their fingers apart. Squeezing silly putty or an exercise band is another method to condition your grip.

Stay mindful of avoiding micro- and macrotrauma to your upper extremities. These overuse conditions develop gradually until they're finally unbearable. For this reason, it's highly recommended that we listen to our bodies and heed what they say. Don't play or work through pain! Just being alert to subtle signs of mild pain can prevent many overuse injuries. Attend to small problems before they manifest into a larger problem.

ARTHRITIS OF THE HANDS & WRIST

EXERCISES/STRETCHES	SETS	REP/TIME	REST
Forearm Flexion & Extension *p. 98*			
Wrist Fold *p. 100*			
Racehorse *p. 101*			
Biceps Curl *p. 94*			
Long Row *p. 86*			
Reverse Fly *p. 72*			
Seated Wrist Stretch *p. 132*			
Inward/Outward Wrist Move *p. 133*			

Arthritis of the wrist and hand can make simple activities painful. The wrist is a complicated joint, with a row of small bones called the carpals that join the two bones of the forearm to form the wrist joint. A capsule of fibrous material as well as ligaments and muscles holds the wrist together. In the case of osteoarthritis, the cartilage that protects the ends of the bone deteriorates, causing the bones to grind against each other.

Wrist issues increase with the degenerative process and can be accelerated by trauma and poor body mechanics. We've seen an increase in wrist problems as typists have moved away from typewriters that required the typist to hit the return lever; that simple motion allowed the hands and wrists to have an active rest period. Also, the prolonged hunched-over position when typing and texting places the neck and upper back in an unhealthy posture, which is why upper body exercises are included in this section.

In rheumatoid arthritis, the synovial membrane becomes inflamed, leading to damage of the bone, cartilage and other structures. Eventually the bones of the joint become poorly aligned and deformed. In the early stages of arthritis of the wrist, mild pain caused by activity can be relieved by rest or splints. However, as the disease progresses, the pain can increase from mild to severe and range of motion is more difficult; If the condition progresses to this level, medical intervention is often required to maintain function. An occupational therapist can teach you to learn how to use adaptive tools to protect your hands, carry bags and perform activities of daily living.

Our hands and opposable thumbs are considered to place humans higher up the evolution ladder. We probably use our hands more than any other joint, so it's not surprising that the incidence of hand/finger issues increases with age. However, with the increased use of texting, hand issues may increase among younger people as well.

TREATMENT OPTIONS

— A comprehensive exam (including X-rays and blood tests) by a physician

— Physical therapy, occupational therapy, corrective exercises

— Conservative measures such as topical lotions, over-the-counter medications, modifying activities, and steroid injections

— Splints

— Input from a medical specialist if these approaches fail

"HANDY" TIPS

1. Be alert to early signs of stiffness and swelling.

2. Seek medical attention early if you suspect hand and finger function is changing. The advice of an occupational therapist is recommended.

3. Accurately describe the symptoms to your physician. If you can't place your palm flat down on a desk, tell your physician.

CARPAL TUNNEL SYNDROME

EXERCISES/STRETCHES	SETS	REP/TIME	REST
Forearm Flexion & Extension *p. 98*			
Seated Wrist Stretch *p. 132*			
Inward/Outward Wrist Move *p. 133*			

Unlike osteoarthritis and rheumatoid arthritis, carpal tunnel syndrome produces numbness and tingling. You may suspect that you have it if you experience weakness or numbness in your hand. Carpal tunnel syndrome also manifests itself when you find it difficult to grip an object or make a fist. The appearance of this syndrome is often seen in people with rheumatoid arthritis, diabetes and poor biomechanics when using a computer keyboard.

The cause of carpal tunnel syndrome is somewhat unknown, although some people say that, in the bygone days of typewriters, we didn't have a high incidence of carpal syndrome because we had to stop for a moment and hit the return lever. An evaluation by medical personnel can usually confirm the diagnosis.

While corrective exercises may help, they're not fully proven. When you begin doing corrective exercises, start with only 1 to 2 reps and be gentle; evaluate how you feel 2 hours post-exercise. If your condition worsens, stop immediately.

TREATMENT OPTIONS

— See a health professional at the first stage of onset

— Splinting

— Injections, surgery

— Physical therapy, occupational therapy, corrective exercises

ELBOW

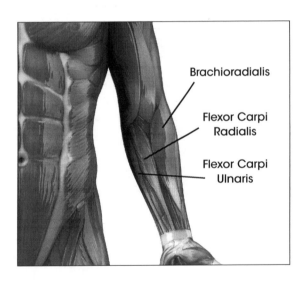

Brachioradialis

Flexor Carpi Radialis

Flexor Carpi Ulnaris

Often, tennis players complain of pain when hitting a backhand stroke. Golfers might experience pain when they hit a shot that digs up a big divot. Elbow problems not only manifest themselves in recreational athletes but also in house painters as well

as carpenters who perform tasks that involve screwing.

The elbow is frequently injured due to overuse. Repetitive activity combined with improper body mechanics contribute to elbow problems. Most people have heard of tennis elbow or Little League elbow, and even manual laborers who use their wrists and hands a great deal develop elbow issues. The pain is usually felt on either the inside or outside of the elbow and sometimes even in the forearm. Excess strain can cause tissue damage or small tears in the elbow tendons.

Conditioning the arm and elbow with corrective exercises in the off-season before you go on the court or golf course will keep you performing pain-free. Learning to properly warm up your body before performing the activity in question can go a long way in keeping you functioning. Evaluating your playing equipment or tools is a prudent idea.

The wrong-sized tennis racquet or relying on a manual screwdriver instead of a power tool could be contributing to your problem.

If you have a tender or painful feeling in your elbow or forearm, take a break from your sport or activity for a while. If it's work related, look for adaptive tools. An occupational therapist is a helpful resource. Seek medical advice to discuss more options

TREATMENT OPTIONS

— Rest

— Application of ice and/or heat

— Medications and/or topical lotions

— Injections

— Braces/supports

— Physical therapy/corrective exercises that consist of stretching and strengthening

EXERCISES/STRETCHES	SETS	REP/TIME	REST
Horizontal Triceps Extension p. 96			
Biceps Curl p. 94			
Triceps Extension p. 97			
Seated Wrist Stretch p. 132			
Inward/Outward Wrist Move p. 133			

SHOULDER

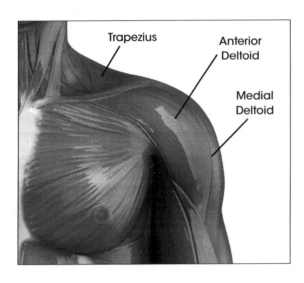

Trapezius

Anterior Deltoid

Medial Deltoid

The shoulder, more accurately called the "shoulder girdle," is a remarkable, complex joint composed of four unique joints/ articulations. It can gently toss an egg back and forth, rock a baby to sleep, hurl a baseball at 90 mph and generate a 100-mph serve in tennis. An engineering marvel, its design

allows for maximum flexibility and function in almost every conceivable direction. This mobility, however, is also why the shoulder joint is so vulnerable to overuse and injuries.

Shoulder pain is reported to occur in 20 percent of the adult population, often persisting for a year or more. Too often people hurt their shoulder because they're not paying attention to how they're using it. If you've had a shoulder injury before, you should be particularly careful. One movement that commonly triggers a shoulder problem is simply reaching too far beyond your "safe" zone. By staying mindful of the green, yellow, red zone concept, you can prevent further shoulder issues. The zones relate to three kinds of shoulder/arm movements: opening your arms (abduction), lifting your arms forward (flexion) and taking your arms backward (extension). Note that each arm/shoulder may have a different comfort zone and that changing hand position can affect mobility in one or both shoulders.

Most people can perform movements in the green zone. When your elbow is in the yellow zone, there is moderate stress on your shoulder; caution should be used in this zone. When you reach into the red zone, the shoulder is unstable and vulnerable to a potential injury. Try to avoid motions in the red zone when possible, especially if you have an injured shoulder.

In addition, avoid the following 13 exercises, which fail the "benefits to risk" index. By staying mindful of these common exercises, you can prevent a shoulder issue.

1. **Lat Pulls** when the bar is pulled down behind the neck or done too quickly and pulled down far below chin level.

2. **Military Presses** done behind the head/neck.

3. **Dumbbell Flys** and **Reverse Flys** done with the arms extremely wide (i.e., in the yellow and red zones).

4. **Bench Presses** with barbell or dumbbells held too wide or with the elbows dipping too far below or behind the bench. Placing the hands in a more neutral grip puts less strain on the shoulder.

5. **Lateral Raises** and **Frontal Raises** done too quickly or lifted higher than shoulder height.

6. **Upright Rows** when the bar is pulled too high.

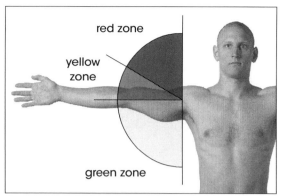

Shoulder abduction zones

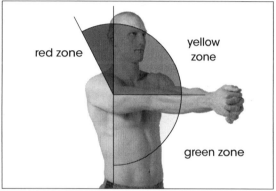

Shoulder flexion zones

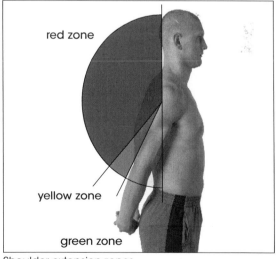

Shoulder extension zones

Staying mindful of the following dos and don'ts will help reduce shoulder issues.

DO

- Separate and lighten loads.

- Lift and carry loads close to your body.

- Take frequent breaks from any repetitious activity.

- When performing activities that are shoulder intensive, such as sweeping or vacuuming, move your whole body by moving your feet and keep your arm tucked in close to your side. Take small steps and keep your back straight.

- Use inexpensive "reachers" or grabber devices to protect your shoulder.

- Practice good posture.

- Rearrange your workstation.

- Alternate the arm you use to carry your briefcase or purse.

- Use caution when your hands are out of your sight.

- Always perform your exercises with proper form.

- Cross-train to avoid overtraining the same muscles in the same manner, day in and day out.

DON'T

- Don't neglect the small supporting muscles of your shoulder joint, such as the rotator cuff muscles.

- Don't slump and let your shoulder round forward.

- Don't work with your arms overhead for prolonged periods.

- Don't lift excessively heavy loads.

- Don't overdo it in activities in which you normally don't participate. Train to play.

---

7. **Shrugs** when done with improper grip width (too wide or too narrow) or when shoulders roll forward and drop quickly. Shrugs when performed with a comfortable weight are ok.

8. **Biceps curls** done on a straight barbell. Instead, use a neutral grip. Dumbbells would be a better choice when doing curls.

9. **Triceps** done with machines or performed with awkward positioning (e.g., French curls).

10. **Wide-grip pull-ups** and **pull-ups** done behind the head.

11. **Repetitive crawl** or **back strokes** when swimming.

12. **Push-ups** when done too wide or done in a manner that strains your shoulder. Push-ups done with hands in a neutral position are best.

13. **Bar dips** done too low or too quickly.

Most shoulder conditions can benefit from these corrective exercises and stretches after a proper warm-up.

- Rotator Cuff Series (page 84)
- Archery Pull (page 93)
- Downward Sword Fighter (page 76)
- Long Row (page 86)
- Reverse Fly (page 72)
- Pull-Down (page 70)
- Elbow Touch (page 114)
- Choker (page 116)
- Shoulder Roll (page 115)
- Shoulder Box (page 115)
- Picture Frame (page 117)

TENDINITIS & BURSITIS IN THE SHOULDER

EXERCISES/STRETCHES	SETS	REP/TIME	REST
Reverse Fly *p. 72*			
Sword Fighter *p. 75*			
Downward Sword Fighter *p. 76*			
Long Row *p. 86*			
Archery Pull *p. 93*			
Pull-Down *p. 70*			
Elbow Touch *p. 114*			
Shoulder Box *p. 115*			
Choker *p. 116*			
Neck Rotation *p. 112*			
Tennis Watcher *p. 112*			

These conditions are closely related and may occur alone or in combination. Tendinitis is inflammation of a tendon. In tendinitis of the shoulder, the rotator cuff and/or biceps tendon become inflamed, usually as a result of being pinched by surrounding structures. The injury may vary from mild inflammation to involvement of most of the rotator cuff. When the rotator cuff tendon becomes inflamed and thickened, it may get trapped under the acromion. Squeezing of the rotator cuff is called impingement syndrome (page 66).

Tendinitis is often accompanied by inflammation of the bursa sacs that protect the shoulder (an inflamed bursa is called bursitis).

Inflammation caused by a disease such as rheumatoid arthritis may cause rotator cuff tendinitis and bursitis. Sports involving overuse of the shoulder and occupations requiring frequent overhead reaching are other potential causes of irritation to the rotator cuff or bursa and may lead to inflammation and impingement.

TREATMENT OPTIONS

The majority of clients who see their medical practitioner about a shoulder problem are there because of tendinitis. Diagnosis of tendinitis and bursitis begins with a medical history and physical examination. X-rays do not show tendons or the bursa but may be helpful in ruling out bony abnormalities or arthritis. Most cases of tendinitis can be successfully treated.

The first step in treating these conditions is to reduce pain and inflammation with rest, ice and anti-inflammatory medicines such as aspirin, naproxen or ibuprofen (such as Advil or Motrin). In some cases, the doctor or therapist will use ultrasound (gentle sound wave vibrations) to warm deep tissues and improve blood flow. Gentle stretching and corrective exercises are recommended and gradually added as you improve. The therapist may suggest a warm pack and gentle active motion, followed by an ice pack. If there's no improvement, the doctor may inject a corticosteroid medicine into the space under your acromion. While steroid injections are a common treatment, they must be used with caution because they may lead to tendon rupture. If there's still no improvement after 6 to 12 months, the doctor may perform either arthroscopic or open surgery to repair damage and relieve pressure on the tendons and bursa.

SHOULDER IMPINGEMENT

EXERCISES/STRETCHES	SETS	REP/TIME	REST
Frontal Raise *p. 73*			
Rotator Cuff—Internal Rotation *p. 84*			
Rotator Cuff—External Rotation *p. 85*			
Shrug *p. 77*			
Elbow Touch *p. 114*			
Choker *p. 116*			
Shoulder Box *p. 115*			
Picture Frame *p. 117*			

Shoulder impingement is a somewhat common chronic condition caused by asking the shoulder joint to do repeated motions day in and day out or trauma, such as falling on the shoulder. You might experience a pinching sensation when raising your arm, pain when sleeping on one side or pain simply when moving your arm.

Seen in people who are extremely hypermobile (their extra flexibility leads to repetitive stress and inflammation), impingement is also increasingly becoming a concern for exercisers and people who perform manual labor or work in a warehouse.

Shoulder impingement is caused by repetitive motions such as those seen in playing tennis or throwing sports such as baseball or softball, and swimming the crawl. Other activities that contribute to shoulder impingement are doing too much overhead work.

TREATMENT OPTIONS

— Rest

— Learning proper biomechanics

— Application of heat and ice

— Physical therapy, corrective exercises

— Medication and medicated pads

— Electrical stimulation or ultrasound treatments

— Steroid injections

— Surgery

ARTHRITIS OF THE SHOULDER JOINT

EXERCISES/STRETCHES	SETS	REP/TIME	REST
Reverse Fly *p. 72*			
Frontal Raise *p. 73*			
Shrug *p. 77*			
Sword Fighter *p. 75*			
Over the Top *p. 116*			
Shoulder Roll *p. 115*			
Picture Frame *p. 117*			

Osteoarthritis of the shoulder is a degenerative condition in which the cartilage deteriorates. This is often the result of chronic wear and tear. However, it can be caused by disease, trauma or infection.

Arthritis of the shoulder is seen earlier in the acromioclavicular joint (formed by the acromion and the clavicle) because it degenerates faster than the glenohumeral joint (the combination of the upper arm bone and the outside area of the scapula). Avoid excessive work/load to the shoulder area. Also, avoid extremes in range of motion in any direction.

CAUSES

— Wear and tear

— Trauma

— Muscle imbalances

— Poor body mechanics when exercising, such as performing deep bench presses and dips

— Overtraining

TREATMENT OPTIONS

— Rest

— Learning proper biomechanics

— Application of heat and ice

— NSAID medications

— Physical therapy, corrective exercises

— Ultrasound, electrical stimulation treatments

— Cortisone injections

ROTATOR CUFF INJURIES

EXERCISES/STRETCHES	SETS	REP/TIME	REST
Downward Sword Fighter *p. 76*			
Rotator Cuff—External Rotation *p. 85*			
Rotator Cuff—Internal Rotation *p. 84*			
Lat Pull-Down *p. 71*			
Long Row *p. 86*			
Sword Fighter *p. 75*			
Shrug *p. 77*			
Over the Top *p. 116*			
Shoulder Roll *p. 115*			
Picture Frame *p. 117*			

Some experts believe that when you move your arm, as many as 26 muscles are engaged. At the gym, people often focus only on the superficial, visible muscles while neglecting crucial, deep muscles that support and provide stabilization to the shoulder joint. The rotator cuff is made up of the SITS muscles: subscapularis, infraspinatus, teres minor and supraspinatus. These muscles share a common tendon.

The most common mechanisms of a rotator cuff injury are separated into either repetitive use or trauma. Rotator cuff tears are seen quite often between the ages of 45 and 65. The most familiar repetitive injuries include poor execution of exercises done in the weight room (e.g., lat pulls behind the neck, improper bench press, upright rowing) or overuse with throwing sports.

TREATMENT OPTIONS

— Rest

— Application of heat and ice

— NSAID medications

— Physical therapy, corrective exercises

— Ultrasound, electrical stimulation treatments

— Cortisone injections

— Surgery

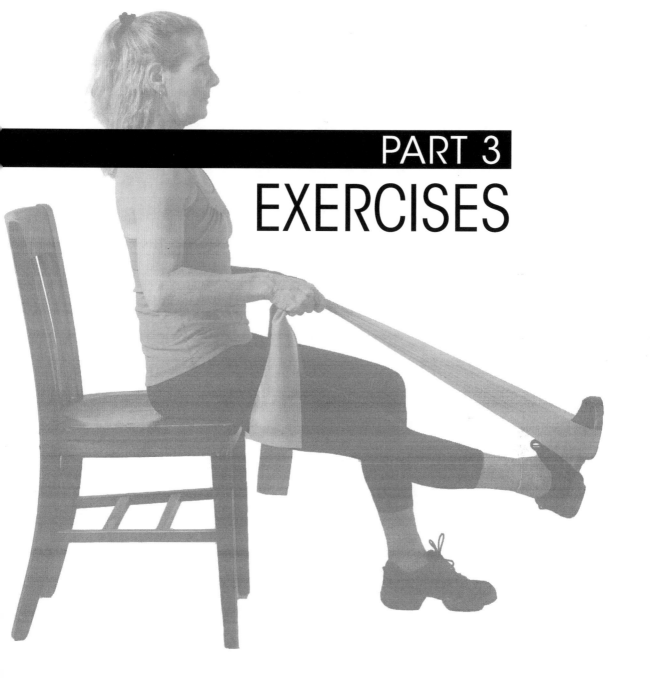

PART 3
EXERCISES

PULL-DOWN

This can be done with one arm or both arms simultaneously, and while sitting or standing.

TARGET: Shoulder, Back

1 Stand upright and hold a band overhead, grasping an end in each hand.

2 Keeping your wrists neutral (don't bend them) and your head and upper back in proper posture, slowly pull both ends of the band downward in front of your shoulders, pausing at shoulder height.

Slowly return to start position.

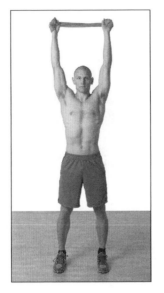

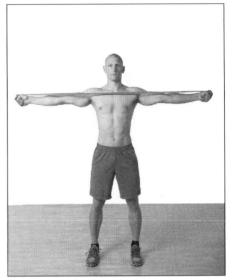

SINGLE-ARM VARIATION: This can also be done with one arm by keeping one arm overhead as the other pulls to the side. Alternate between left and right arms.

LAT PULL-DOWN

Always double-check that the band won't come loose when you apply force. Don't allow the band to snap off and injure you.

TARGET: Latissimus Dorsi, Arms

1 Secure the band firmly to the top of a door or something tall and grab an end in each hand. Step backward until the band provides your desired resistance. Sit on the floor or in a chair, with your arms straight and angled upward and back mostly straight.

2 Keeping your elbows close to your ribs, slowly pull the band down toward your chest. Hold for 1–2 seconds.

Slowly release your arms to the start position.

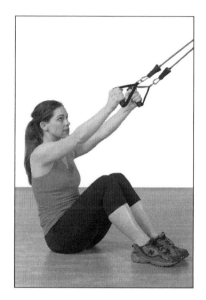
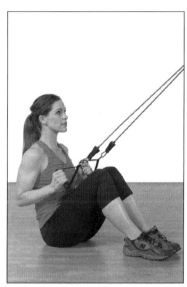

REVERSE FLY

This can be done with one arm or both arms simultaneously, and while sitting or standing. As you improve, reduce the slack in the band to increase resistance.

TARGET: Upper Back, Shoulder (posterior deltoid)

1 Stand upright and hold a band in front of your chest, grasping it in each hand. Extend your arms straight out in front of you. Adjust your grip until you have the desired resistance.

2 Keeping your arms parallel to the floor, your wrists neutral (don't bend them) and your head and upper back in proper posture, slowly open your arms out to the sides.

Slowly return to start position.

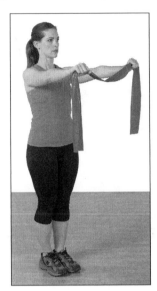
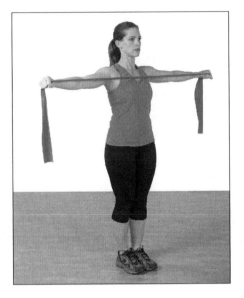

SINGLE-ARM VARIATION: You can also move one arm at a time, keeping the other arm extended in front of your chest. Perform all your reps with one arm before switching arms, or alternate arms.

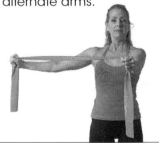

FRONTAL RAISE

This can be done with one arm or both arms simultaneously, and while sitting or standing.

TARGET: Shoulder

1 Stand in the middle of the band and grasp an end in each hand. Place your arms alongside your body with your palms facing your thighs. Adjust your grip on the band until it provides the desired resistance.

2 Keeping your arms straight, slowly raise your arms forward no higher than shoulder height.

Slowly lower to start position.

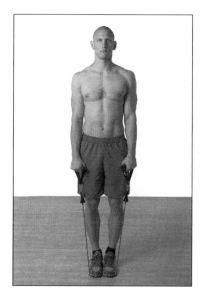
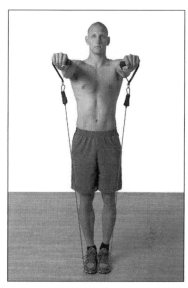

LATERAL RAISE

This can be done with one arm or both arms simultaneously, and while sitting or standing.

TARGET: Shoulder

1 Stand in the middle of the band and grasp an end in each hand. Place your arms alongside your body with your palms facing your body. Adjust your grip on the band until it provides the desired resistance.

2 Keeping your arms straight, slowly raise your arms to the sides no higher than shoulder height.

Slowly lower to start position.

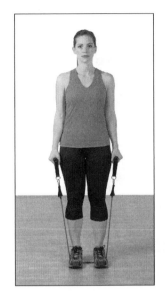

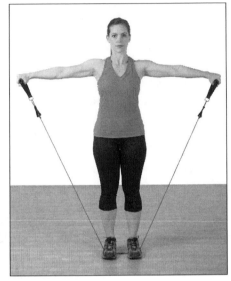

SINGLE-ARM VARIATION:
This can also be done with one arm. Do one arm first before switching, or alternate between left and right arms.

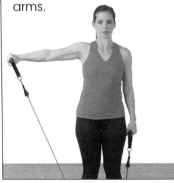

SWORD FIGHTER

As you improve, reduce the slack in the band to increase resistance.

TARGET: Shoulder (posterior deltoid)

1 Stand with proper posture and secure an end of the band on your right hip with your right hand. Then grasp the band with your left hand at a location that provides the desired resistance.

2 Keeping your left arm straight, slowly pull the band diagonally upward across your body as if pulling out a sword.

Controlling the speed, slowly return to start position.

Repeat, then switch sides.

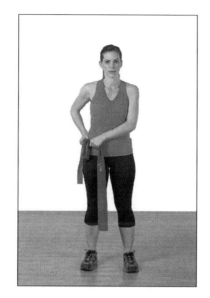 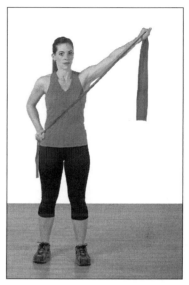

DOWNWARD SWORD FIGHTER

TARGET: Upper Back

1 Stand with proper posture and hold one side of the band in your left hand slightly above your head with your thumb pointing down. Grasp the band with your right hand at a location that provides adequate resistance.

2 Slowly pull your right hand diagonally down past your right hip.

Slowly allow the band to return to start position.

Repeat, then switch sides.

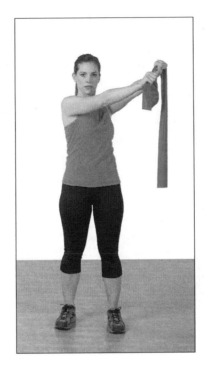
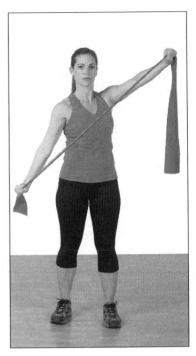

SHRUG

TARGET: Trapezius

1 Stand in the middle of the band with knees softly bent and grasp an end in each hand. Your hands should be in front of your hips, palms facing your body. Adjust your grip on the band until you have your desired resistance.

2 Keeping your arms straight, slowly "shrug" your shoulders to your ears. Hold 1–2 seconds.

Slowly return to start position.

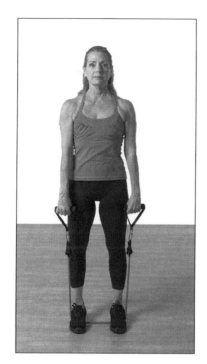
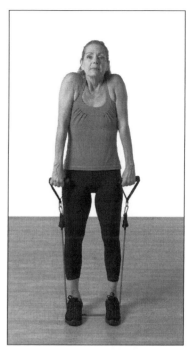

BAND PUSH-UP

This is an advanced exercise.
TARGET: Chest, Triceps

1 Placing the band around your upper back and then under each hand, assume a plank position with your arms straight, hands directly under your shoulders, and legs extended behind you so that your body forms a straight line. Adjust the band to keep the band snug when in the down position.

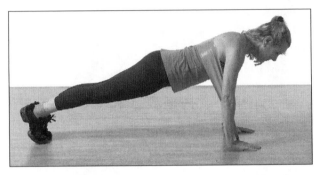

2 While maintaining an aligned posture, slowly lower your chest to the floor. Keep your body straight; don't sag in the middle.

Extend your arms and return to start position.

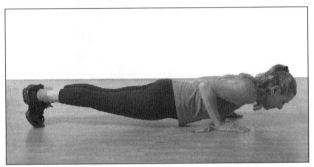

MODIFICATION: This can also be done from your knees.

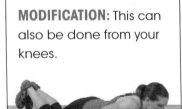

HORIZONTAL CHEST PRESS

CAUTION: *This is an advanced shoulder exercise.*

TARGET: Chest

1 Sit or stand with proper posture and place the band behind your mid-upper back. Grasp the band in each hand at a point of adequate resistance in front of your shoulders.

2 Keeping your wrists neutral (don't bend them) and your head and upper back in proper posture, slowly press both ends of the band forward. Pause when your arms are extended in front of you.

Slowly return to start position.

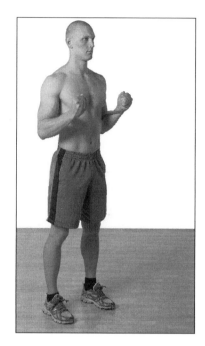
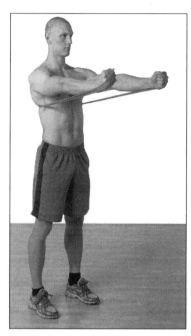

INCLINE CHEST PRESS

CAUTION: *This is an advanced shoulder exercise.*

TARGET: Upper Shoulder, Chest

1 Sit or stand with proper posture and place the band behind your mid-upper back. Grasp the band in each hand at a point of adequate resistance in front of your shoulders.

2 Keeping your wrists neutral (don't bend them) and your head and upper back in proper posture, slowly press both ends of the band forward and upward at a 45-degree angle. Pause when your arms are extended in front of you.

Slowly return to start position.

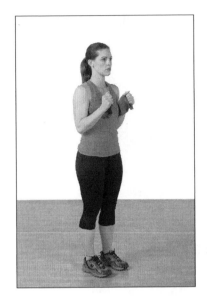 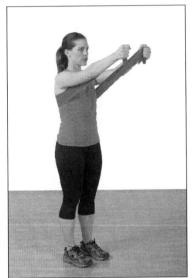

FLY

CAUTION: *This is an advanced shoulder exercise.*
TARGET: Shoulder, Chest

1 Sit or stand with proper posture and place the band behind your mid-upper back. Grasp the band in each hand in front of your shoulders and open your arms out to the sides.

2 Keeping your wrists neutral (don't bend them) and your head and upper back in proper posture, slowly bring your hands toward each other in front of your chest.

Keeping tension in your arms, slowly return to start position.

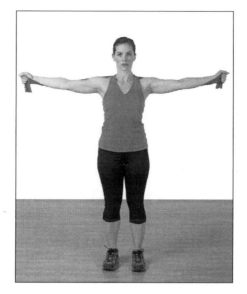

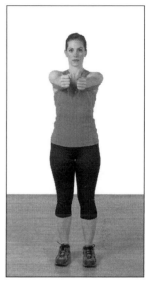

INCLINE VARIATION:
Extend the arms upward at a 45-degree angle before taking them out to the sides.

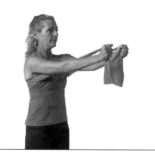

CHEST FLY

Always double-check that the band won't come loose when you apply force. Don't allow the band to snap off and injure you.

TARGET: Chest, Shoulder

1 Attach the band securely to a door using band straps. With your back to the door, grasp an end of the band in each hand with your arms extended to your sides, palms facing forward.

2 Keeping your arms somewhat straight, bring your arms together in front of your chest, palms facing each other.

Slowly return to start position.

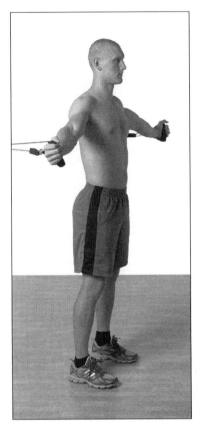 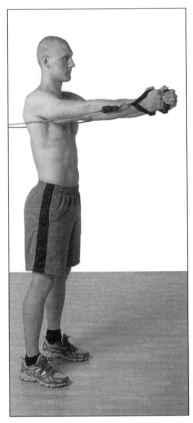

SHOULDER PRESS

This can be performed while sitting in a chair or standing.

CAUTION: *This is an advanced shoulder exercise.*

TARGET: Shoulder

1 Sit or stand with proper posture and place the band behind your mid-upper back and under your armpits. Grasp the band in each hand in front of your shoulders at a location that provides adequate resistance.

2 Keeping your wrists neutral (don't bend them) and your head and upper back in proper posture, slowly press both ends of the band up toward the ceiling. Pause when your arms are extended.

Slowly return to start position.

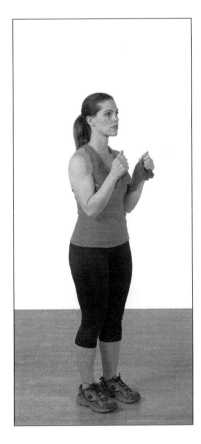
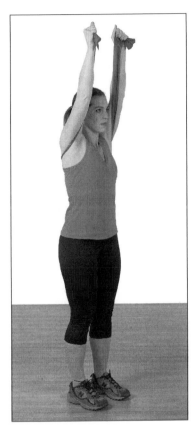

ROTATOR CUFF—INTERNAL ROTATION

For a better grip, tie a small knot in the band and then place the band between your ring finger and middle finger with your thumb pointed up. Always double-check that the band won't come loose when you apply force. Don't allow the band to snap off and injure you. You may roll up a small towel and place it alongside your rib cage and next to the arm of the affected shoulder for better biomechanical placement of the shoulder joint.

TARGET: Rotator Cuff

1 Attach the band securely to a stable object (e.g., door knob) at belly button height. With the right side of your body facing the anchor, grasp the band with your right hand, palm facing inward, place your right elbow next to your ribs, and bend your elbow 90 degrees. Then move sideways from the anchor until you're at a distance that provides adequate resistance.

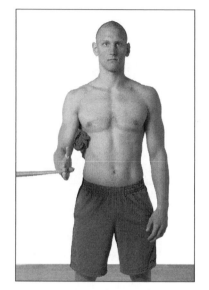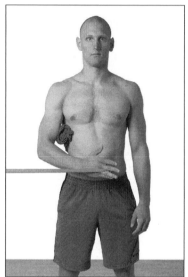

2 Keeping your shoulders back and torso engaged, slowly and mindfully move your right hand to cover your belly button.

Slowly and carefully return to start position.

Repeat, then switch sides.

ROTATOR CUFF—EXTERNAL ROTATION

Heavy resistance isn't important here. Double-check that the band won't come loose when you apply force. Don't allow the band to snap off and injure you. You may roll up a small towel and place it alongside your rib cage and next to the arm of the affected shoulder for better biomechanical placement of the shoulder joint.

TARGET: Rotator Cuff

1 Attach the band securely to a stable object (e.g., door knob) at belly button height. With the left side of your body facing the attachment point, grasp the band with your right hand. For a better grip, tie a small knot in the band and then place the band between your ring and middle finger with your thumb pointed up. Your right palm should face your body and your right elbow should be bent 90 degrees and next to your ribs. Adjust your distance until you get your desired resistance.

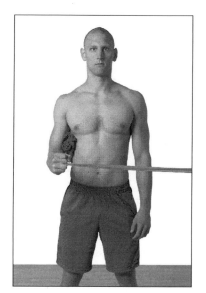 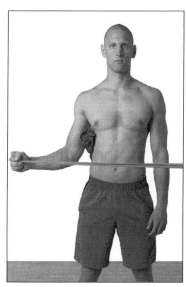

2 Keeping your shoulders back and torso engaged, slowly and mindfully move your right hand out to the side (do not to go out too far).

Slowly and carefully return to start position.

Repeat, then switch sides.

LONG ROW

Always double-check that the band won't come loose when you apply force. Don't allow the band to snap off and injure you.

TARGET: Back, Arm

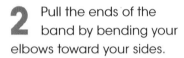

1 Attach the band securely to the bottom of a door or any other stable object. Sit on the floor facing the door then extend your legs straight. Grasp an end of the band in each hand at a location that provides adequate resistance. Keep your torso at roughly 90 degrees.

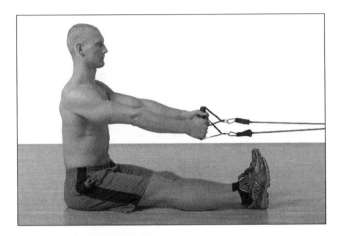

2 Pull the ends of the band by bending your elbows toward your sides.

Slowly allow your arms to return to start position.

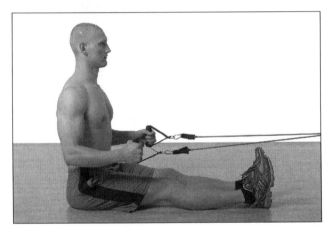

VARIATION: This can also be done without an attachment. Simply loop the middle of the strap around both feet.

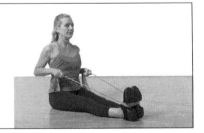

TORSO CURL

TARGET: Abdominals

1 While sitting, place the band under your tailbone. Run it under your spine as you lie on your back with your knees bent and feet flat on the floor. Grasp the top of the band with both hands; the weight on your tailbone should secure the other end.

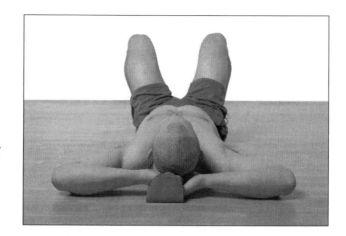

2 Tucking your chin to your chest while pressing your lower back into the floor, slowly curl up. Hold.

Return to start position.

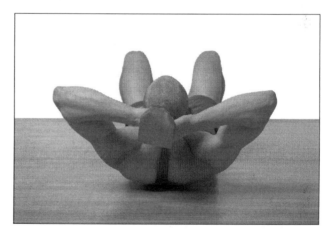

CHAIR SIT-UP

Note that core exercises performed from the floor are superior to this exercise. This exercise is offered for those who cannot perform such core exercises.

TARGET: Abdominals

1 Sit in a chair with proper posture and place the band behind the upper portion of your chair. Grasp an end of the band in each hand near your shoulders. Adjust your grip on the band until you have your desired resistance.

2 Slowly bend your torso forward. Pause.

Slowly return to start position.

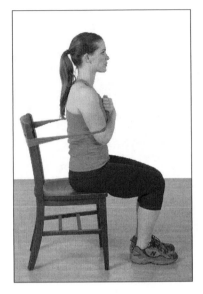 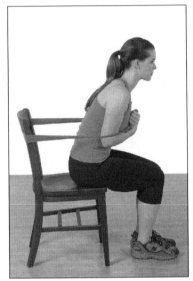

PELVIC LIFT

TARGET: Quads, Gluteals, Para-Spinal Back Muscles

1 Lie on your back. Place the band over your hips and secure it firmly by holding each end of the band with your hands.

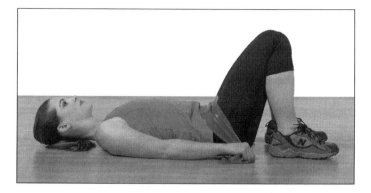

2 Slowly lift your hips to a comfortable height. Engage your butt muscles; don't use momentum. Hold for 1–2 seconds.

Return to start position.

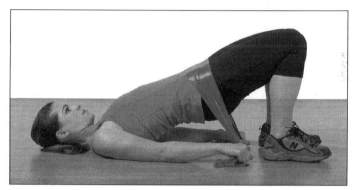

REVERSE WOOD CHOP

TARGET: Core

1 Assume a fairly wide staggered stance and step on the band with your left foot. With both hands, grasp the band close to hip height at a point that provides ideal resistance.

2 Rotate your torso diagonally upward to the right, extending your arms upward.

Slowly return to start position. Repeat, then switch sides.

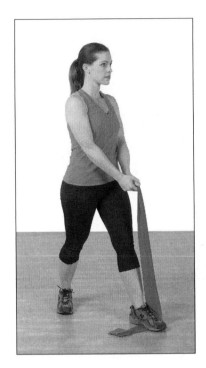
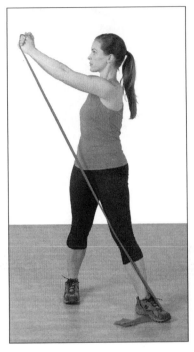

SIDE BEND

CAUTION: *Be careful if you have arthritis of the spine.*
TARGET: Core

1 Stand with your feet shoulder-width apart and place a band under your right foot. Grasp the band near your right hip with your right hand.

2 Lean your body to the left.

Return to start position. Repeat, then switch sides.

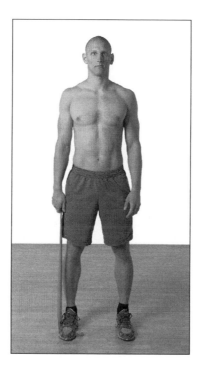
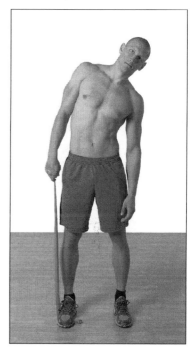

TORSO ROTATION

Always double-check that the band won't come loose when you apply force. Don't allow the band to snap off and injure you.

TARGET: Core

1 Secure the band to a door with the proper strap so that the band is at chest height. While standing with your right side to the door, grab the band with both hands and move away from the door until your arms are fully extended. Stand with your feet shoulder-width apart.

2 Slowly twist to the left and hold for 1–2 seconds.

Return to start position.

Repeat, then switch sides.

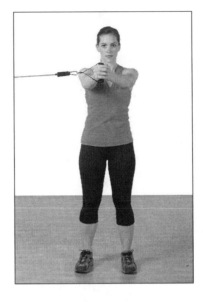
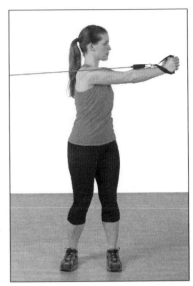

ARCHERY PULL

TARGET: Upper Back, Biceps

1 Sit or stand with proper posture. Hold one end of the band in your left hand and extend your left arm straight out to the side. With your right hand, grasp the band near your left elbow or shoulder at a location that provides proper resistance.

2 Pull your right arm across your chest, drawing your elbow to your right side.

Slowly return to start position.

Repeat, then switch sides.

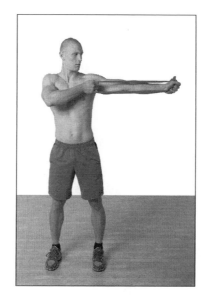
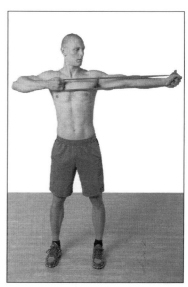

BICEPS CURL

TARGET: Biceps

1 Stand in the middle of the band and hold an end of the band in each hand with your palms facing forward. Adjust your grip on the band until you have your desired resistance.

2 Keeping your elbows close to your ribs, bend your arms to slowly bring your palms toward your shoulders.

Slowly lower your arms.

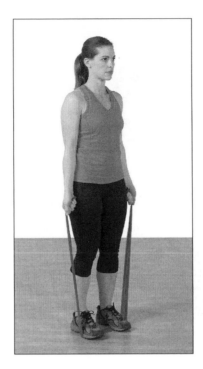 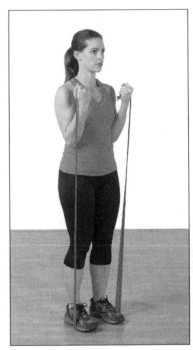

REVERSE CURL

TARGET: Biceps, Forearm

1 Stand in the middle of the band and hold an end of the band in each hand with your palms facing your body. Adjust your grip on the band until you have your desired resistance.

2 Keeping your elbows close to your ribs, bend your arms to slowly bring your knuckles toward your shoulders.

Slowly lower your arms.

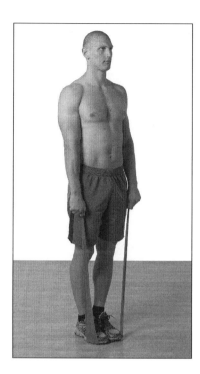
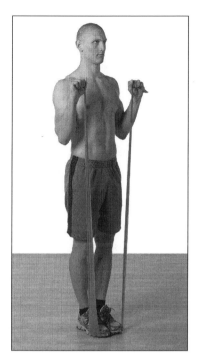

HORIZONTAL TRICEPS EXTENSION

TARGET: Triceps

1 Sit or stand with proper posture and grasp the band with both hands approximately shoulder-width apart and at chest height. Lift your elbows out to the sides, keeping your arms parallel to the floor.

2 Keeping your right hand in place, slowly extend your left arm out to the side.

Slowly return to start position. Alternate between left arm and right arm.

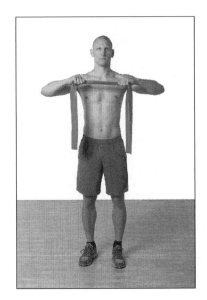
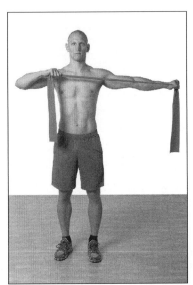

DOUBLE-ARM VARIATION: Perform the motion with both arms at the same time.

TRICEPS EXTENSION

TARGET: Triceps

1 Stand with proper posture. Drape the band over your right shoulder and secure the band by placing your left hand on top of it. Bend your right elbow roughly 90 degrees and place it next to your ribs. With your right hand, grasp the band at a location that provides your desired resistance.

2 Without using momentum, slowly extend your right arm and hold for 1–2 seconds.

Slowly return your arm to a 90-degree position.

Repeat, then switch sides.

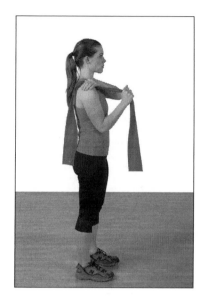 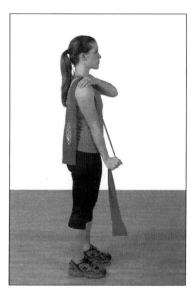

FOREARM FLEXION & EXTENSION

To reduce stress on your wrist, allow the band to run between your ring and middle fingers.

TARGET: Wrist, Forearm

1 Sit on the edge of the chair and step securely on the band. Place your forearm on the same thigh as the hand you will use. Roll up one end of the band into your hand and place the palm up. Adjust the band until you have your desired resistance.

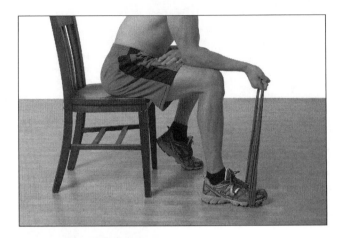

2 Slowly curl (flex) your palm toward your body. Pause.

Slowly return to start position.

Repeat, then switch sides.

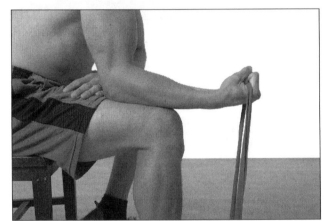

3 Now turn your palm down. Slowly curl (flex) the back of the hand upward toward your body. Pause.

4 Slowly return to start position.

Repeat, then switch sides.

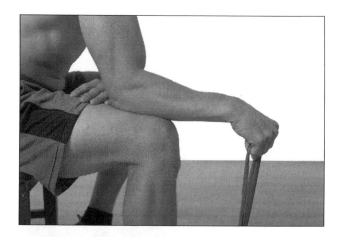

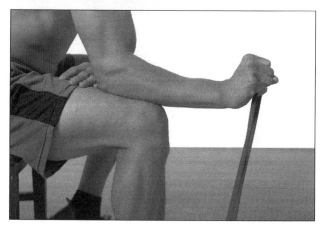

WRIST FOLD

TARGET: Forearm

1 Sit or stand with proper posture and extend your arm while holding one end of the band.

2 Turn your palm up and grab more band in your hand.

3 Turn your palm down and grab more band, balling it up in your hand as you go. Continue rotating your hand until the band is inside your palm. Once the band is inside your hand, squeeze it firmly 10 times.

Repeat, then switch sides.

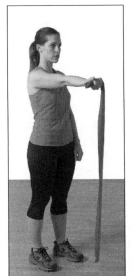
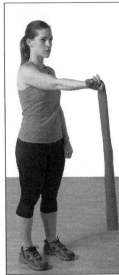
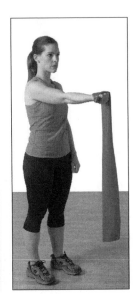

RACEHORSE

TARGET: Hand, Forearm

1 Sit or stand with proper posture and extend your arm while holding one end of the band.

2-3 Quickly grab some band and pull it into the palm of your hand while squeezing the band. Continue until the entire band is inside your palm. Once the band is inside your hand, squeeze it firmly 10 times.

Repeat, then switch sides.

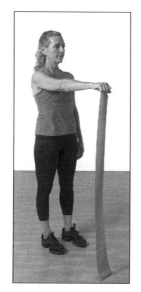
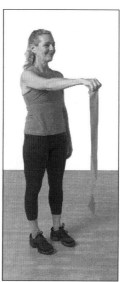
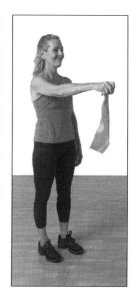

SQUEEZER

You can also try doing this with an object in both hands.

TARGET: Hand, Forearm

1 Sit with proper posture in a stable chair.

2 Hold a small, soft, squeezable object in one hand and extend that arm straight out in front of you. Keep your other arm by your side. Slowly squeeze the object and hold for 1–2 seconds.

Repeat until the hand has done a comfortable number. Switch hands and repeat.

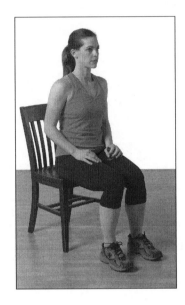 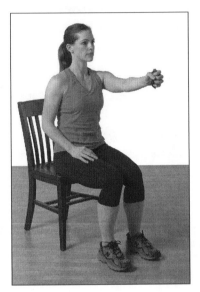

> **VARIATION:** Try this on something more difficult to squeeze, like a tennis ball.

GAS PEDAL

TARGET: Calf

1 Sit with proper posture. Place one foot on the floor and extend the other leg straight out in front of you. Wrap the band around the ball of your foot once to keep it in place.

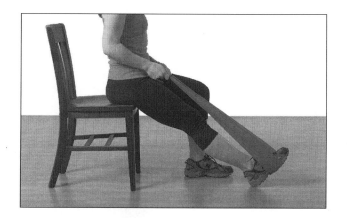

2 Slowly point your foot, keeping tension in the band.

Return your foot to neutral.

Repeat, then switch sides.

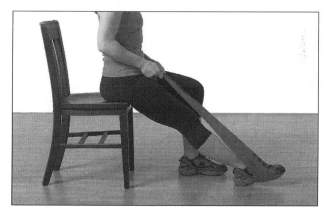

SEATED LEG PRESS

TARGET: Thighs

1 Sit with proper posture in the middle of a chair. Place one foot on the floor and extend the other leg straight out in front of you. Wrap the band once around the ball of the foot of the other leg to keep it in place. Slowly bring your knee in toward your chest.

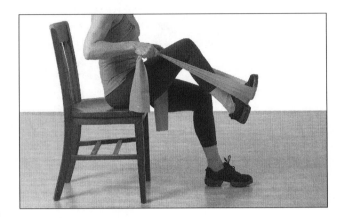

2 Extend your leg, making sure not to lock your knee.

Return to start position.

Repeat, then switch sides.

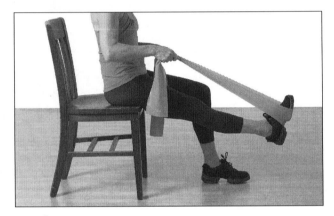

LEG CURL

If balance is an issue, you may want to stand near a secure location for assistance.

CAUTION: *Be careful of hamstring cramps.*

TARGET: Hamstrings

1 Place a circular band under one foot and wrap the band around the other ankle, or tie one end of the band around the ankle. Wrap the band so that it provides resistance through the full range of motion.

2 Maintaining neutral spine position, slowly curl the leg that has the band around the ankle halfway up. Control the motion in both directions—don't allow the band to determine the speed. Hold for 1–2 seconds.

Slowly lower the leg to start position.

Repeat, then switch sides.

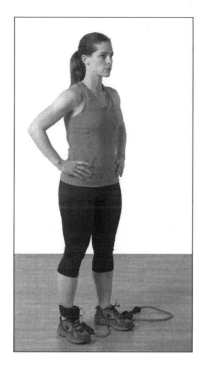
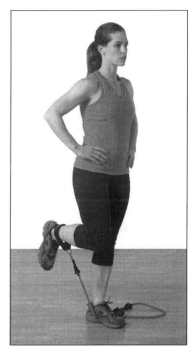

SQUAT

TARGET: Quadriceps

1 Stand with your feet hip-width apart on the band. Grasp an end of the band in each hand at a place that offers your desired resistance.

2 Keeping your back in neutral position, squat down halfway, adjusting the resistance as necessary. Don't allow your knees to extend past your toes. Pause.

Return to start position.

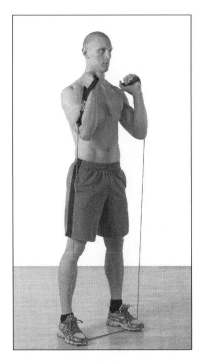
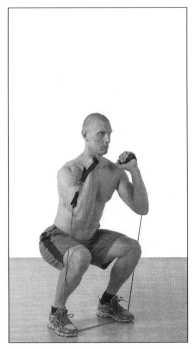

SQUAT SHUFFLE

TARGET: Quadriceps

1 While standing with your feet about 6 inches apart, wrap a circular band around your legs at mid-thigh or tie a band around both thighs.

2 Squat either a quarter- or halfway down and then take 4 steps to the right. Don't allow your knees to extend past your toes.

3 Now take several steps to the left. Continue stepping to the left and right.

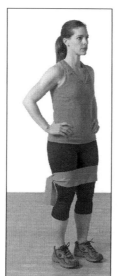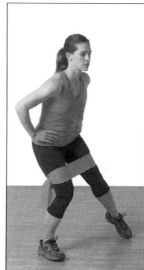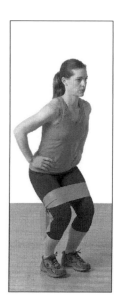

FORWARD LUNGE

Use a lighter band that's extra long for this more-advanced move.

TARGET: Quadriceps

1 Stand in the middle of the band with your left foot and hold on to the band with each hand at a location that provides adequate resistance. Slide your right foot backward.

2 Attempt to lower your right knee to the floor if possible, otherwise just go as low as is comfortable, using the left leg for stability. You should feel an increase in resistance in the left leg as you come upright.

Repeat, then switch sides.

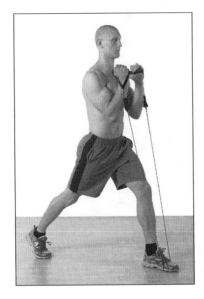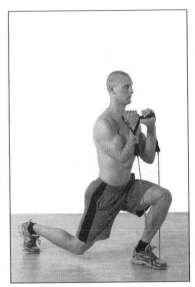

SIDE LUNGE

TARGET: Iliotibial Band

1 While standing with your feet about 6 inches apart, wrap a circular band around your legs at mid-thigh or tie a band around both thighs.

2 Take 4 steps to the right—do not overstride—and then take 4 steps to the left. Continue stepping to the left and right.

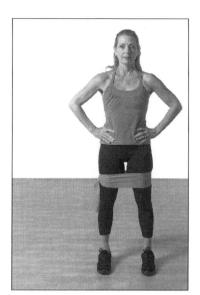 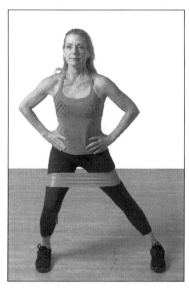

LEG ABDUCTION & ADDUCTION

If you have balance issues, hold onto something for stability. Always double-check that the band won't come loose when you apply force. Don't allow the band to snap off and injure you.

CAUTION: *Avoid this exercise if you have hip problems.*

TARGET: Iliotibial Band, Glutes, Abductor Muscles, Adductor Muscles, Groin

1 Secure the band firmly to the bottom of a door or similar solid object. Attach the ankle cuff to your ankle and then position yourself perpendicular to the door. It should provide resistance through the full range of motion. Position the strapped ankle far away from the door.

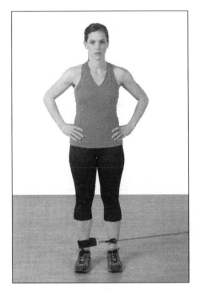
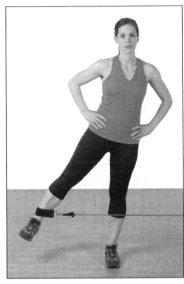

2 Slowly move your leg to the side a comfortable distance.

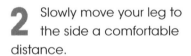

3 Slowly lower the leg to start position. Repeat, then switch sides.

4 Turn 180 degrees so that the strap is now on the leg closest to the door. Slowly move the strapped leg in front of and across your body.

Slowly return the leg to start position. Repeat, then switch sides.

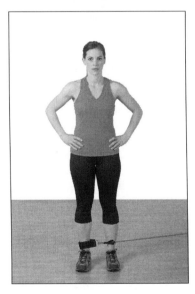
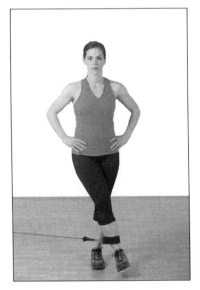

REVERSE LEG EXTENSION

Always double-check that the band won't come loose when you apply force. Don't allow the band to snap off and injure you.

TARGET: Gluteus Maximus, Hamstrings

1 Attach one end of the band to a secure object such as a door or sturdy chair and the strap to the right ankle. Face the door/object; use it for balance if necessary.

2 Keeping your leg straight, slowly extend your leg backward to engage your butt muscles. Hold 1–2 seconds.

Slowly return to start position. Repeat, then switch sides.

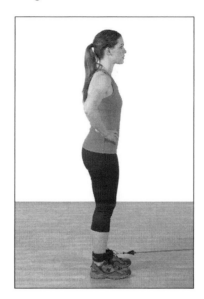 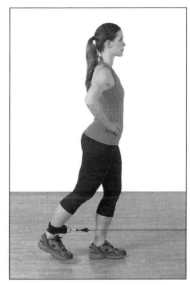

NECK ROTATION

TARGET: Neck

1 Sit or stand with proper posture. Inhaling slowly through your nose, look to your left as far as you can without feeling discomfort.

2–3 Exhale and slowly trace your collarbone with your chin until you're looking to your right.

Inhale and repeat to the other side.

Repeat as desired.

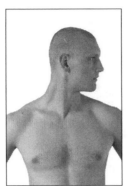
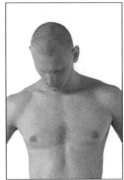
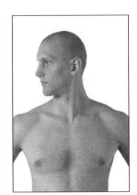

TENNIS WATCHER

TARGET: Neck

1 Sit or stand with proper posture. While inhaling slowly through your nose, look to your left as far as you can without feeling discomfort. Exhale slowly through your lips and hold this position for a moment, feeling the stretch.

2 Now inhale slowly through your nose and look slowly to the right. Exhale slowly through your lips and hold this position for a moment, feeling the stretch.

Repeat as desired.

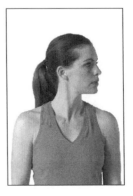
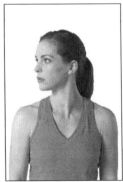

SOUP CAN

TARGET: Deltoids, Rotator Cuff

1 Stand with proper posture, your arms at your side and your palms facing back.

2 Inhale deeply through your nose and bring both arms slightly forward as you raise them out to the sides, keeping your palm facing back. Raise your arms no higher than shoulder level.

Exhale as you lower your arms to start position.

Repeat as desired.

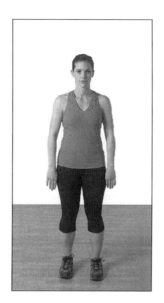
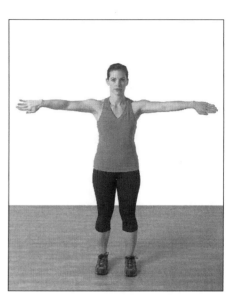

ELBOW TOUCH

You can also try this stretch sitting with proper posture in a stable chair.

TARGET: Chest, Shoulder Retractor

1 Stand with proper posture. Place your hands on your shoulders, elbows pointing forward.

2 Slowly bring your elbows together in front of your body.

3 Bring your elbows back and squeeze your shoulder blades together. Hold for a moment, focusing on opening up your chest.

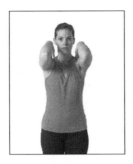
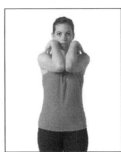
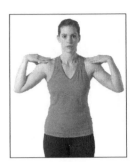

Bring your elbows back to start position and repeat as desired.

VARIATION: Once you've done Step 1, draw circles with your elbows.

SHOULDER BOX

TARGET: Trapezius

1 Stand with proper posture. Inhaling deeply through your nose, slowly lift up your shoulders.

2 Now pull your shoulders back and squeeze the shoulder blades together and down.

Exhaling through your lips, drop your shoulders and return to start position.

Repeat as desired.

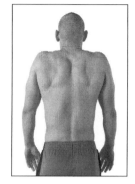 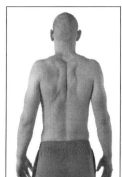

SHOULDER ROLL

TARGET: Trapezius

1 Sit or stand with proper posture. Inhale slowly and deeply through your nose. Exhaling through your nose, roll your shoulders forward, attempting to touch your shoulders together.

2 Now inhale and focus on squeezing your shoulder blades together, moving your shoulders back and opening up your chest.

Repeat as desired.

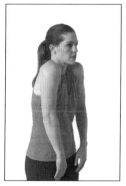 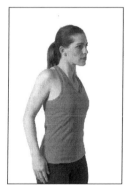

OVER THE TOP

TARGET: Deltoids, Rotator Cuff

1 Sit or stand with proper posture. Raise your left arm and place your hand on your back, over your left shoulder. Place your right hand on your left elbow and gently press your left arm down your back as far as feels comfortable. Hold the position for a comfortable moment.

Switch sides and repeat.

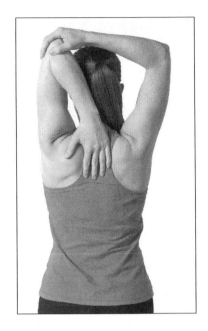

ISOMETRIC VARIATION: Press your left arm down as you push your left elbow up into your hand. Hold this position for a comfortable moment, remembering to breathe. Then release and allow your hand to slide a little farther down your back.

CHOKER

TARGET: Deltoids, Rotator Cuff

1 Sit or stand with proper posture. Place your right hand on your left shoulder. Place your left hand on your right elbow and gently press your right elbow toward your throat. Hold for a comfortable moment.

Switch sides and repeat.

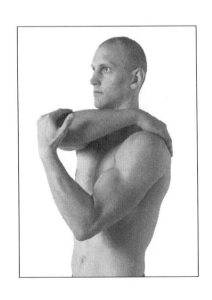

ISOMETRIC VARIATION: Press your right elbow into your left hand. Hold for a comfortable moment, remembering to breathe. Then release to reach the right hand a little farther back.

PICTURE FRAME

Remember not to let your lower back arch.

TARGET: Deltoids

1 Sit or stand with proper posture. Place your
right hand on your left elbow and your left
hand on your right elbow.

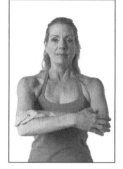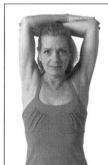

2 Slowly lift your arms overhead, raising them as
high as feels comfortable. Hold the position
for a moment. You're now framing your face in a
picture frame created by your arms—smile.

Repeat as desired.

MAD CAT

TARGET: Total Body

1 Rest on your hands and knees.

2 Draw your belly button in, causing your back
to round. Inhale deeply.

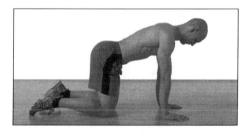

Now exhale and slowly relax your body to the start
position.

Repeat as desired.

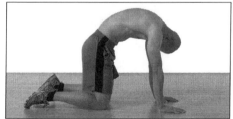

LONG BODY STRETCH

For this stretch, try listening to some relaxing music.
TARGET: Total Body

THE POSITION: Lie on a mat, with your head on a pillow if needed. Focus on breathing slowly in and out through your nose. Reach your arms as far back as is comfortable. Lengthen your legs as far as is possible. Try to make your body as long as possible while breathing in a comfortable fashion. Remember to focus on your breath.

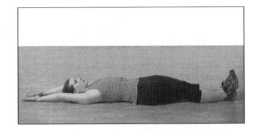

SIDE BEND

You can also try this stretch while standing with proper posture.
CAUTION: *Be careful if you have lower back pain.*
TARGET: Torso, Deltoids

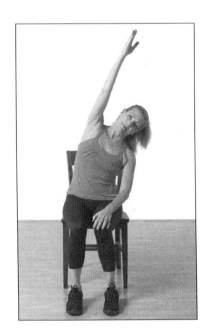

THE POSITION: Sit with proper posture in a stable chair. Raise your right arm over your head to a comfortable height. Inhale deeply through your nose. Now exhale through your lips and slowly and carefully lean to the left. Once you've leaned over enough to feel a gentle stretch along the right side of your body, hold this position for a comfortable moment.

Switch sides and repeat.

MODIFICATIONS: If your shoulder is stiff, place your hand on top of your head. If raising your arm at all is very painful, just leave your arm alongside your body.

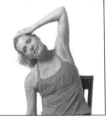

SINGLE KNEE TO CHEST

TARGET: Lower Back, Gluteus Maximus

1 Lie on a mat and, if needed, place a pillow under your head. Bend your knees and place both feet flat on the floor. Loop a strap behind the back of your right leg and hold one side of the strap in each hand.

2 Gently pull the straps to bring the knee toward your chest. Hold this stretch for a comfortable moment.

Release the knee, switch sides and repeat.

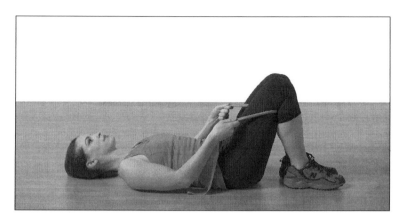

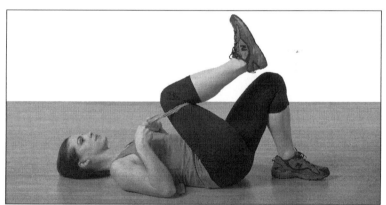

VARIATION: This can also be done by bringing both knees to the chest at the same time.

INTERMEDIATE VARIATION: This can also be done using just the hands to bring in the knee.

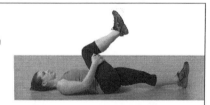

ADVANCED VARIATION (ABOVE): Extend one leg straight on the floor and bring the other knee to your chest.

PIRIFORMIS STRETCH

The piriformis muscle is a deep-lying muscle in the gluteal region, through which the sciatic nerve passes. When the piriformis is too tight, it can cramp the sciatic nerve, causing the symptoms of sciatica.

TARGET: Piriformis, Lower Back

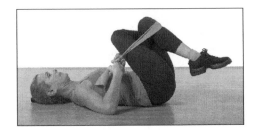

THE POSITION: Lie on a mat with your knees bent and your feet flat on the floor. Cross your right knee on top of your left knee. Loop a strap around both legs and pull your knees in toward your chest. Stop when tension occurs. Hold this position for a comfortable moment, focusing on the sensation of the stretch.

Switch sides and repeat.

> **VARIATION:** Use only your hands to pull your knees in.

FIGURE 4

TARGET: Hamstrings

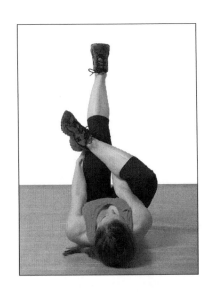

THE POSITION: Lie on a mat with your knees bent and your feet flat on the floor. Place your right ankle on top of your left knee. Wrap both hands around your left leg and bring your knee and ankle to your chest. Now straighten your left leg toward the ceiling as much as is comfortable. Focus on inhaling and exhaling fully and hold this stretch for a comfortable moment.

Switch sides and repeat.

QUAD STRETCH

CAUTION: *Avoid this exercise if you have poor balance. STOP if you notice undue compression in your knee or experience any lower back discomfort. If you feel a cramp coming on, do a hamstrings stretch.*

TARGET: Quadriceps

1 Stand with proper posture facing a chair and loop a strap around your right ankle.

2 Bring your right heel toward your butt. Keep both knees as close together as possible. Gently pull your heel closer to your bottom, using the back of the chair for balance if necessary. Hold this stretch for a comfortable moment.

Switch sides and repeat.

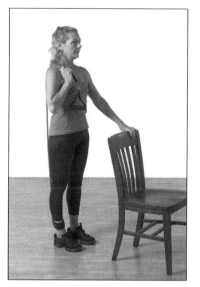
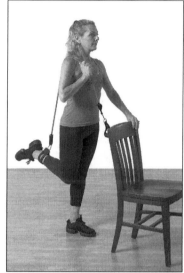

INTERMEDIATE VARIATION (LEFT): Try this without the strap by grabbing your foot with your hand.

ADVANCED VARIATION (RIGHT): Try this without the chair and with the strap in one arm, raising your free arm toward the ceiling.

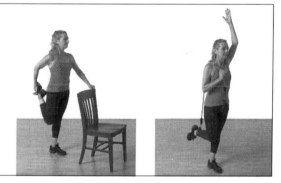

STRAIGHT-LEG STRETCH

TARGET: Hamstrings, Lower Back

1 Sit at the edge of a stable chair and place both feet flat on the floor. Position a strap around the sole of the right foot and hold an end of the strap in each hand.

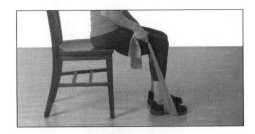

2 Inhale deeply through your nose and straighten your right leg. Now exhale through your lips and attempt to straighten your right leg as far as is comfortable. Hold this position for a comfortable moment.

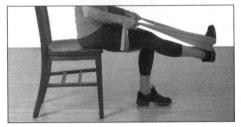

> **VARIATION:** This can also be performed while lying on your back, with the strap positioned around the sole of your foot. Your other leg can be extended along the floor or bent with your foot on the ground.

INNER THIGH STRETCH

TARGET: Inner Thigh

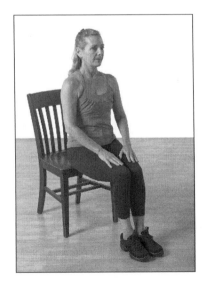
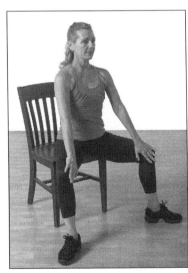

THE POSITION: Sit at the edge of a stable chair and place both feet flat on the floor. Spread your legs apart and point your knees and toes out to the sides 45 degrees. Place your hands on the insides of your thighs and gently push your legs a little wider. Hold this stretch for a comfortable moment.

Repeat as desired.

ILIOTIBIAL BAND STRETCH

CAUTION: *If you've been advised by your doctor or therapist not to cross your legs, do not do this exercise.*

TARGET: Iliotibial Band

THE POSITION: Stand with proper posture next to a chair on your left side. Cross your left leg in front of your right leg. Raise your right arm up overhead and lean to the left, gently pressing your right hip outward to the right. Use the chair for balance. Hold this stretch for a comfortable moment.

Switch sides and repeat.

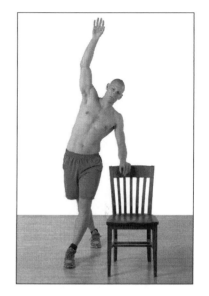

> **MODIFICATION:** If your shoulders are tight, just place your hand on your hips.
>
> **VARIATION:** If balance is not an issue, try this without the chair.

THE BUTTERFLY

TARGET: Inner Thigh, Lower Back

THE POSITION: Sit on the ground and place the soles of your feet together. Gently allow your knees to drop to the floor. Loop a strap around your feet and gently pull yourself forward, not down. Hold this stretch for a comfortable moment.

Repeat as desired.

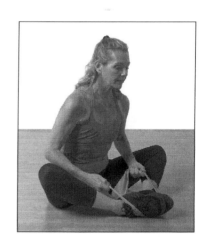

PRETZEL

TARGET: Iliotibial Band

1 Sit at the edge of a stable chair. Cross your right knee over your left.

2 Reach both hands around the top of the right knee. Gently twist to the right while pulling the knee toward the midline of your body. Hold this stretch for a comfortable moment.

Switch sides and repeat.

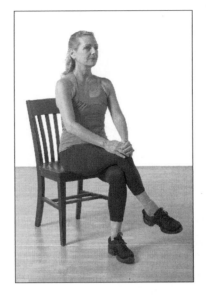
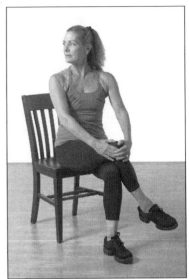

VARIATION: This exercise can also be done while sitting on the floor with your legs straight out in front of you. Bend your right knee and place your right foot on the outside of your left leg, as close to the left knee as possible. Then gently twist to the right, as you look left.

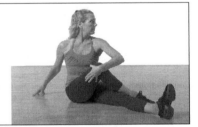

STANDING HIP FLEXOR

TARGET: Hip Flexor

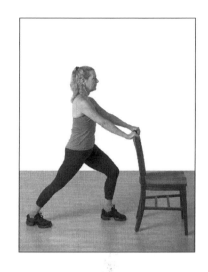

THE POSITION: Stand behind a chair and place your hands on the back of it. Slide your right leg back a comfortable distance. Keeping your rear heel down, gently tuck your tailbone under and press your hips forward. Hold this stretch for a comfortable moment, focusing on feeling the stretch in the upper leg/hip region rather than in the calf area.

Switch sides and repeat.

REAR CALF STRETCH

TARGET: Calf

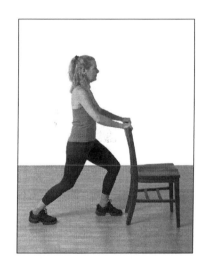

THE POSITON: Stand behind a chair, placing both hands on the back of it. Keeping the heel down, slide your right leg as far back as you can. Bend your left knee until the desired stretch is felt in the calf area. Hold this stretch for a comfortable moment.

Switch sides and repeat.

DROP-OFF STRETCH

CAUTION: *Only do this exercise if you're fairly flexible. Do not force anything, do not do this move if you have a history of Achilles heel injury, and do not do if you're unsure of your balance.*

TARGET: Calf

1 Stand behind a chair, using the back for support. Place your right foot on a block.

2 Gently and slowly lower your right heel until the desired stretch is felt in the calf area. Hold this stretch for a comfortable moment, using the chair for balance if necessary.

Switch sides and repeat.

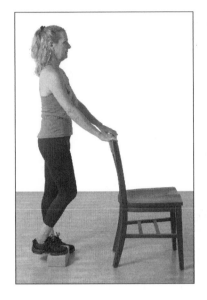 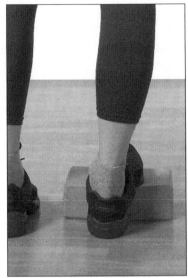

REAR CALF STRETCH WITH STRAP

TARGET: Calf

1 Stand with proper posture, holding an end of the strap in each hand. Step your left foot forward and loop the strap around the ball of the foot.

2 Keeping your heel on the floor, gently pull your toes up until you feel the desired stretch in your calf. Hold for a comfortable moment.

Switch sides and repeat.

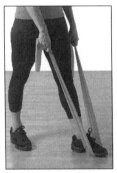 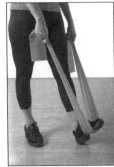

GAS PEDAL STRETCH

CAUTION: *Don't force your toes in either direction. Be aware that your calf may cramp when extending your toes. Be careful not to tip the chair over.*

TARGET: Ankle

1 Sit at the edge of a stable chair. Extend your right leg straight out in front of you and lift it off the ground. Point your toes up and hold for several seconds.

2 Extend your toes away from you and hold for several seconds.

Repeat a comfortable number of times and then switch sides.

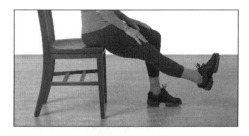

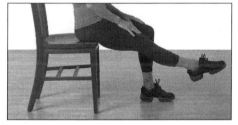

HEEL RAISE/HEEL DROP

TARGET: Ankle

1 Sit at the edge of a stable chair and place a block under the balls of your feet.

2 Keeping the balls of your feet on the block, raise your heels and hold the stretch for several seconds.

3 Drop your heels and hold the stretch for several seconds.

Repeat a comfortable number of times.

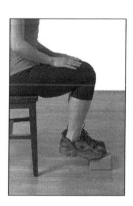

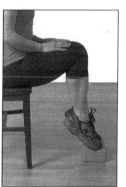

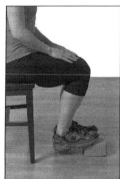

ANKLE CIRCLE

TARGET: Ankle

1 Sit at the edge of a stable chair. Extend your right leg straight out in front of you and lift it off the ground.

2–3 Keeping your leg stationary (using your hands for support, if necessary), point your toes and draw several circles with your foot in both directions.

Switch sides and repeat.

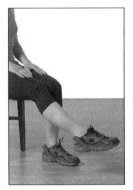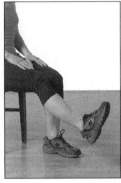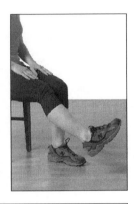

ANKLE WRITING VARIATION: Point your toes and write your address and phone number with your foot. Switch sides and repeat.

SELF-ROM

TARGET: Ankle

1 Sit at the edge of a stable chair. Cross your left ankle on top of your right knee and gently grasp your left foot with your right hand.

2 Slowly use your hand to gently move your foot in comfortable circles as well as forward and backward.

Switch sides and repeat.

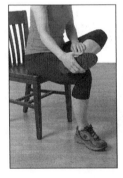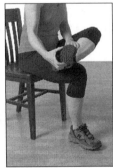

ANKLE ROLLER

If you don't have a foam roller, you can also use a rolling pin, a frozen orange juice container (good for icing sore feet) or a can of soup.

TARGET: Ankle

1–2 Sit at the edge of a stable chair and place both feet on the floor, directly below your knees. Place a roller under the arch of your right foot. Slowly move your foot back and forth over the roller.

Switch sides and repeat.

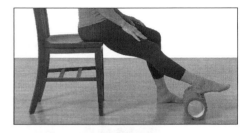

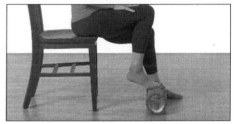

FINGER SPREADER

TARGET: Hand, Forearm

1 Sit with proper posture in a stable chair. Rest your hands on your thighs with your palms down. Pinch your fingers and thumb together.

2 Now separate all fingers and thumb as far apart as possible.

Turn your palms up and repeat.

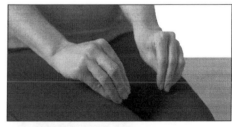

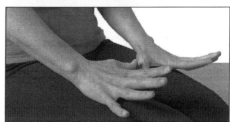

FINGER TAP

TARGET: Hand, Forearm

1 Sit at the edge of a stable chair. Rest your hands on your thighs with your palms turned up.

2 Touch your little finger to your thumb then progress through each finger until you reach your index finger.

3 Now turn your palms down and repeat the exercise.

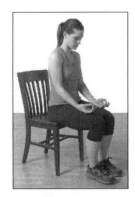
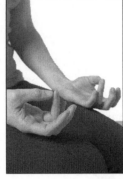
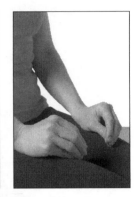

FINGER BASE TAP VARIATION:
Touch the thumb to the base of your little finger, then progress through each finger until you reach the index finger. Now turn your palms down and repeat the exercise.

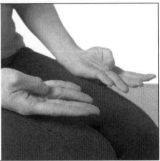

V-W STRETCH

TARGET: Hand

1 Sit with proper posture in a stable chair. Rest your hands on your thighs with your palms down. Squeeze all your fingers together.

2 Separate one finger at a time, starting with the little finger, then the ring finger, until you've separated all your fingers. Squeeze your fingers together and repeat the exercise.

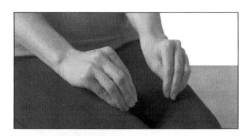

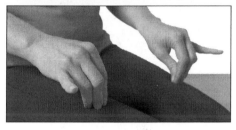

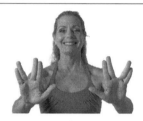

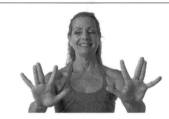

VARIATION: Increase the challenge by holding your arms straight out in front of you. Instead of just separating your fingers, try to make a V and W.

TO MAKE A V: Spread your little finger and ring finger away from your index finger and middle finger.

TO MAKE A W: Put your ring finger and middle finger together and separate the little finger and index finger from the group.

SEATED WRIST STRETCH

TARGET: Wrist, Forearm

1 Sit in a stable chair. Rest your forearms on your thighs so that your wrists hang off. Your hands are in a loose fist. Slowly lift your knuckles toward the ceiling and hold 1–2 seconds.

2 Slowly lower your knuckles toward the floor and hold 1–2 seconds.

Repeat as desired.

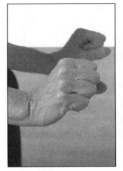
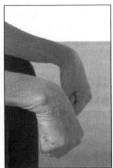

STANDING WRIST STRETCH

TARGET: Wrist, Forearm

1 Stand with proper posture. Extend your right arm in front of you to shoulder height, with your palm facing forward and fingers pointing toward the ceiling.

2 Gently pull your fingers back with your left hand until a desired stretch is felt under your wrist. Hold the stretch for several seconds.

Repeat as desired then switch sides.

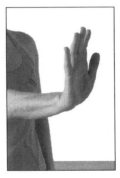
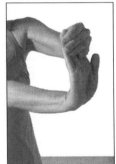

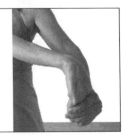

VARIATION: Try doing the exercise with the fingertips pointing down.

INWARD/OUTWARD WRIST MOVE

TARGET: Wrist, Forearm

1 Sit with proper posture in a stable chair. Rest your fists on your thighs with your thumbs pointing up toward the ceiling.

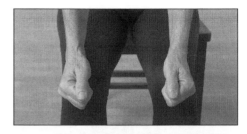

2 Slowly turn your fists so that your thumbs point inward.

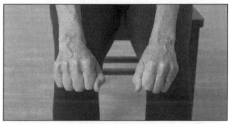

3 Slowly turn your fists so that your thumbs point outward.

Repeat as desired.

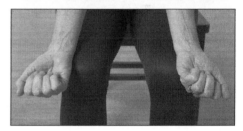

INDEX

Achilles tendon issues, 31–32

ACL injuries, 44–45

Acute phase, of rehabilitation, 11

Aging, and physiological systems, 22

Ankle Circle, 128

Ankle Roller, 129

Ankles/feet, 26–27; Achilles tendons, 31–32; arthritis, 28–29; corrective routines, 28–32; illustration, 26; sprains, 25, 30; stretching exercises, 127–29

Archery Pull, 93

Arms: exercises, 94–102. *See also* Elbows; Hands/wrists; Shoulders

Arthritis: ankles/feet, 28–29; hands/wrists, 55–56; hip, 37; knee, 47–48; shoulder, 67

Back/torso, 49–50; corrective routines, 50; exercises, 86–93; illustration, 49; stretches, 117–20, 122–23

Band Push-Up, 78

Benefits-to-risk ratio, 20, 61

Biceps Curl, 94

Blood pressure, 12, 16

Breathing, 12, 16

Bursa sacs, 35, 43, 64

Bursitis, 25; knee, 43; legs/hips, 35–36; shoulder, 64–65

The Butterfly, 123

Carpal tunnel syndrome, 57

Chair Sit-Up, 88

Chest Fly, 82

Choker, 116

Chronic orthopedic issues, 22–25

Color, of resistance bands, 8

Comfort zone, for shoulder exercises, 60–61

Cooper, Ken, 4

"Corrective exercise" concept, 23

Corrective resistance training: equipment, 8–9; exercises, 70–133; FAQs, 15–16; overview, 12–20; process, 10–14; program design, 18–20; routines, 22–68; stretching, 112–33; tips, 12

Corrective routines, 22–68. *See also specific body issues and/or conditions*

Corrective stretching exercises, 112–33
Corrective training tips, 12

Degenerative joint disease (DJD), 24. *See also* Arthritis
Deterioration, of bands, 9
"Dose and response" concept, 19
Downward Sword Fighter, 76
Drop-Off Stretch, 126

Elbow Touch, 114
Elbows, 58–59; corrective routines, 59; illustration, 58
Equipment, 8–9
Exercise bands. *See* Resistance bands
Exercises, 70–133; arm/hand, 94–102; back/torso, 86–93; leg/hip, 103–11; shoulder, 70–85; stretching, 112–33

Fallen arches, 31
FAQs, 15–16
Feet. *See* Ankles/feet
Figure 4, 120
Finger Spreader, 129
Finger Tap, 130
Flat feet, 31
Flat resistance bands, 8–9
Fly, 81
Forearm Flexion & Extension, 98–99
Forward Lunge, 108
Frequency, of training, 16
Frontal Raise, 73
Functional fitness, 2
Functional phase, of rehabilitation, 12–13

Gas Pedal, 103
Gas Pedal Stretch, 127
Green zone concept, 60–61
Groin strain, 38

Handles, on bands, 8, 9
Hands/wrists, 53–54; arthritis, 55–56; carpal tunnel syndrome, 57; corrective routines, 55–57, exercises, 98–99, 101–102; illustration, 53; stretching, 129–33
Heel Raise/Heel Drop, 127
Hip bursitis, 35–36
"Hip hurter" exercises, 34
Hip joint, 33–34
Hips. *See* Legs/hips
Horizontal Chest Press, 79
Horizontal Triceps Extension, 96

Iliotibial (IT) band, 39
Iliotibial band fasciitis, 39–40
Iliotibial Band Stretch, 123
Impingement, shoulder, 66
Incline Chest Press, 80
Inner Thigh Stretch, 122
Inward/Outward Wrist Move, 133

Joint health, 10, 17. *See also specific joints* (Elbows; Knees; *etc.*)

Kinetic chain, 26
Knees, 41–42; arthritis, 47–48; bursitis, 43; corrective routines, 43–48; illustration, 41; ligament injuries, 44–45; meniscus injuries, 46

Lat Pull-Down, 71
Lateral Raise, 74
Latex allergies, 8
Leg Abduction & Adduction, 110
Leg Curl, 105
Legs/hips, 33–34; arthritis, 37; bursitis, 35–36; corrective routines, 35–40; exercises, 103–11; groin strain, 38; iliotibial band fasciitis, 39–40; illustration, 33; stretches, 121–26. *See also* Ankles/feet; Knees
Long Body Stretch, 118

Long Row, 86
Lower back. *See* Back/torso

Mad Cat, 117
Medical clearance, 3, 12. *See also specific health issues*
Meniscus injuries, 46
"Mind body" approach, 5

Neck, 51–52; corrective routines, 52; illustration, 51; stretches, 112
Neck Rotation, 112

Orthopedic issues, chronic, 22–25
Osteoarthritis (OA), 24, 47–48. *See also* Arthritis
Over the Top, 116
Overpronation, 31

Pain, and rehabilitation, 11–12
Pelvic Lift, 89
Picture Frame, 117
Piriformis Stretch, 120
Posture, 12, 13–14
Prehabilitation stage, 11
Pretzel, 124
Progress, tracking, 19
"Progressive load" concept, 6
Pull-Down, 70
"Pulled muscles." *See* Strains
PVC pipe, as handle, 8, 9

Quad Stretch, 121

Racehorse, 101
Rear Calf Stretch, 125
Rear Calf Stretch with Strap, 126
Recovery phase, of rehabilitation, 11
Red zone concept, 60–61
Rehabilitation, 2–20; equipment, 8–9; exercises, 70–133; FAQs, 15–16; history, 4–5; phases, 11–13; process, 10–14; program design, 18–20; routines, 22–68. *See also specific body issues and/or conditions*
Reps, 15
Resistance bands, 2, 6–7; safety, 9; selection, 8–9; storage, 9
Resistance-training. *See* Corrective resistance training
Resting, between sets, 15–16
Reverse Curl, 95
Reverse Fly, 72
Reverse Leg Extension, 111
Reverse Wood Chop, 90
Rotator cuff injuries, 68
Rotator Cuff—External Rotation, 85
Rotator Cuff—Internal Rotation, 84
Routines. *See* Corrective routines

"Safe" zone concept, 60–61
Safety issues, 9. *See also* Medical clearance
Sciatica, 49, 120
Seated Leg Press, 104
Seated Wrist Stretch, 132
Self-ROM, 128
Sets, 15
Shoes, 27, 28
Shoulder, 60–63; arthritis, 67; bursitis, 64–65; comfort zone, 60–61; corrective routines, 63–68; do's and don'ts, 62; exercises, 70–85; exercises to avoid, 61–63; illustration, 60; impingement, 66; rotator cuff, 68; stretches, 113–18; tendinitis, 64–65
Shoulder Box, 115
Shoulder Press, 83
Shoulder Roll, 115
Shrug, 77
Side Bend, 91
Side Bend (stretch), 118
Side Lunge, 109
Single Knee to Chest, 119

Soup Can, 113

Sprained ankles, 30

Sprains, 25, 30

Squat, 106

Squat Shuffle, 107

Squeezer, 102

Standing Hip Flexor, 125

Standing Wrist Stretch, 132

Storage, of bands, 9

Straight-Leg Stretch, 122

Strains, 25

Stretching, 12, 16; corrective exercises, 112–33

Surgical tubing, 6–7

Sword Fighter, 75

Tendinitis, 25; shoulder, 64–65

Tennis Watcher, 112

Torso. *See* Back/torso

Torso Curl, 87

Torso Rotation, 92

Training tips, 12

Triceps Extension, 97

Trochanteric bursitis (hip bursitis), 35–36

Tubular resistance bands, 9

2-hour rule, 19

V-W Stretch, 131

Warming up, 12, 16

Water exercise, 24

Women, and knee injuries, 44

Wrist Fold, 100

Wrists. *See* Hands/wrists

Yellow zone concept, 60–61

ACKNOWLEDGMENTS

A special thanks goes out to Kelly Reed for her vision along, with the behind-the-scenes team at Ulysses Press. A special shout out goes to Lily Chou for making sense of my writing, as well as the rest of the editorial team, Claire Chun and Lindsay Tamura.

Another thought of appreciation goes to Rapt Productions and the models Bryan Ausinheiler, Caitlin Halferty and Toni Silver.

Last but not least, thank you to my son Chris for his insights and critical suggestions on content of the book, and Margaret, my wife of 40 years, for dealing with me. Let's not leave out my other son Kevin for reminding me that laughter is the best medicine and that a hearty laugh works your abdominal muscles better than sit-ups. Thanks to all my former students who taught me life is too short to be cranky and that how you make a person feel is most important.

ABOUT THE AUTHOR

Dr. Karl Knopf is the author of numerous fitness books, including *Stretching for 50+*, *Foam Roller Workbook*, *Resistance Band Workbook*, and *Make the Pool Your Gym*. Dr. Karl, as his students used to call him, has been involved in the health and fitness of older adults and the disabled for more than 40 years. During this time he has worked in almost every aspect of the industry, from personal training and therapy to consultation.

While at Foothill College, Karl was the coordinator of the Adaptive Fitness Technician Program and Life Long Learning Institute. He taught disabled students and undergraduates about corrective exercise. In addition to teaching, Karl developed the "Fitness Educators of Older Adults Association" to guide trainers of older adults. Currently Karl is a director at the International Sports Science Association and is on the advisor board of PBS's *Sit and Be Fit* show.

In his spare time he has spoken at conferences, authored many articles, and written numerous books on topics ranging from water workouts to fitness therapy. He was a frequent guest on both radio and print media on issues pertaining to senior fitness and the disabled.

Made in the USA
Middletown, DE
16 November 2022